www.bma.org.uk/library

ABC OF BURNS

KT-430-859

WITHDRAWN FROM LIBRARY

BMA LIBRARY
BRITISH MEDICAL ASSOCIATION

WITHDRAWN FROM LIBRARY

BRITISH MEDICAL ASSOCIATION

0520948

ABC OF BURNS

Edited by

SHEHAN HETTIARATCHY

*Specialist registrar in plastic and reconstructive surgery,
Pan-Thames Training Scheme, London*

REMO PAPINI

*Consultant and clinical lead in burns, West Midlands Regional Burn Unit,
Selly Oak University Hospital, Birmingham*

and

PETER DZIEWULSKI

*Consultant burns and plastic surgeon, St Andrew's Centre for Plastic Surgery and Burns,
Broomfield Hospital, Chelmsford*

WITHDRAWN FROM LIBRARY
BMA LIBRARY
BRITISH MEDICAL ASSOCIATION

BMJ
Books

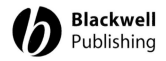
Blackwell
Publishing

© 2005 by Blackwell Publishing Ltd
BMJ Books is an imprint of the BMJ Publishing Group, used under licence

Blackwell Publishing, Inc., 350 Main Street, Malden, Massachusetts 02148-5020, USA
Blackwell Publishing Ltd, 9600 Garsington Road, Oxford OX4 2DQ, UK
Blackwell Publishing Asia Pty Ltd, 550 Swanston Street, Carlton, Victoria 3053, Australia

The right of the Authors to be identified as the Authors of this Work has been asserted in accordance with
the Copyright, Designs and Patents Act 1988.

All rights reserved. No part of this publication may be reproduced, stored in a retrieval system, or
transmitted, in any form or by any means, electronic, mechanical, photocopying, recording or otherwise,
except as permitted by the UK Copyright, Designs and Patents Act 1988, without the prior written
permission of the publisher.

First published 2005

Library of Congress Cataloging-in-Publication Data
ABC of burns / edited by Shehan Hettiaratchy, Remo Papini, and Peter Dzicwulski.
    p. ; cm.
  Includes bibliographical references and index.
  ISBN 0-7279-1787-0
  1. Burns and scalds. 2. Burns and scalds—Treatment. 3. Burns and scalds—Patients—Rehabilitation.
  [DNLM: 1. Burns—classification. 2. Burns—psychology. 3. Burns—therapy. 4. Emergency Treatment—
methods. 5. Reconstructive Surgical Procedures—methods. Wo 704 A1366 2005] I. Hettiaratchy, Shehan.
II. Papini, Remo. III. Dziewulski, Peter.

  RD96.4.A225 2005
  617.1′1—dc22

                                                                                          2004022733

ISBN-13: 978 0 7279 1787 4
ISBN-10: 0 7279 1787 0

A catalogue record for this title is available from the British Library

Cover is courtesy of Jerry Mason/Science Photo Library

Set by BMJ Electronic Production
Printed and bound in Spain by GraphyCems, Navarra

Commissioning Editor: Eleanor Lines
Development Editors: Sally Carter/Nick Morgan
Production Controller: Kate Charman

For further information on Blackwell Publishing, visit our website:
http://www.blackwellpublishing.com

The publisher's policy is to use permanent paper from mills that operate a sustainable forestry policy, and
which has been manufactured from pulp processed using acid-free and elementary chlorine-free practices.
Furthermore, the publisher ensures that the text paper and cover board used have met acceptable
environmental accreditation standards.

Contents

Contributors   vii

Preface   ix

1   Introduction   1
      Shehan Hettiaratchy, Peter Dziewulski

2   Pathophysiology and types of burns   4
      Shehan Hettiaratchy, Peter Dziewulski

3   First aid and treatment of minor burns   7
      Jackie Hudspith, Sukh Rayatt

4   Initial management of a major burn: I—overview   10
      Shehan Hettiaratchy, Remo Papini

5   Initial management of a major burn: II—assessment and resuscitation   13
      Shehan Hettiaratchy, Remo Papini

6   Management of burn injuries of various depths   16
      Remo Papini

7   Intensive care management and control of infection   19
      Mark Ansermino, Carolyn Hemsley

8   Burns reconstruction   23
      Juan P Barret

9   Rehabilitation after burn injury   26
      Dale Edgar, Megan Brereton

10   Psychosocial aspects of burn injuries   29
      Shelley A Wiechman, David R Patterson

11   Burns in the developing world and burn disasters   32
      Rajeev B Ahuja, Sameek Bhattacharya

12   When we leave hospital: a patient's perspective of burn injury   35
      Amy Acton

Index   39

Contributors

Amy Acton
Executive director of the Phoenix Society for Burn Survivors, East Grand Rapids, MI, USA

Rajeev B Ahuja
Head of the Department of Burns, Plastic, Maxillofacial, and Microvascular Surgery, Lok Nayak Hospital and associated Maulana Azad Medical College, New Delhi, India

Mark Ansermino
Paediatric anaesthesiologist, British Columbia's Children's Hospital, Vancouver, Canada

Juan P Barret
Consultant plastic and reconstructive surgeon, St Andrew's Centre for Plastic Surgery and Burns, Broomfield Hospital, Chelmsford

Sameek Bhattacharya
Specialist in the Department of Burns, Plastic, Maxillofacial, and Microvascular Surgery, Lok Nayak Hospital and associated Maulana Azad Medical College, New Delhi, India

Megan Brereton
Occupational therapist in the Upper Limb Rehabilitation Unit, Royal Perth Hospital, Perth, Australia

Peter Dziewulski
Consultant burns and plastic surgeon, St Andrew's Centre for Plastic Surgery and Burns, Broomfield Hospital, Chelmsford

Dale Edgar
Senior physiotherapist, in Burns and Plastic Surgery, Royal Perth Hospital, Perth, Australia

Carolyn Hemsley
Specialist registrar in infectious diseases and microbiology, John Radcliffe Hospital, Oxford

Shehan Hettiaratchy
Specialist registrar in plastic and reconstructive surgery, Pan-Thames Training Scheme, London

Jackie Hudspith
Clinical nurse lead, Burns Centre, Chelsea and Westminster Hospital, London

Remo Papini
Consultant and clinical lead in burns, West Midlands Regional Burn Unit, Selly Oak University Hospital, Birmingham

David R Patterson
Professor in the Department of Rehabilitation Medicine, University of Washington School of Medicine, Seattle, USA

Sukh Rayatt
Specialist registrar in plastic and reconstructive surgery, West Midlands Training Scheme, Birmingham

Shelley A Wiechman
Acting assistant professor in the Department of Rehabilitation Medicine, University of Washington School of Medicine, Seattle, USA

Preface

Burns are one of the most devastating injuries that can be experienced. Burns are an assault on the physical, psychological and physiological aspects of the patient, affecting all ages and all populations around the world. The sequelae of burns are long-lasting; scars, both physical and emotional, may soften but do not disappear. The only way to treat such a diverse injury is to have an integrated, multi-disciplinary team approach. This allows all aspects of the patient's changing needs to be addressed, so that a reasonable recovery can be achieved.

The aim of this ABC series is to provide the non-specialist with an overview of burn care. It is hoped that the initial chapters will be helpful in the management of acute burns and that the later chapters will provide an insight into the more long-term management of these patients. We have endeavoured to provide a voice for all members of the burns team and also provide a perspective from around the world. In the last chapter the most important person involved in burn injuries speaks; the patient. The patient's perspective is one that is easily overlooked but it is by far and away the most important.

There are many different ways to manage burn injuries and the methods we describe are not "the" way of managing burns, just "a" way. It is how we manage our burn patients but readily accept that others use different techniques with similar results. What we are trying to do is provide some kind of framework of burn care for the non-specialist, not perform an exhaustive treatise.

We would like to thank our reviewers, Rob Sheridan and Helena Elkington, for their excellent critiques and guidance. We would also like to thank all at the BMJ, in particular Eleanor Lines; we have often needed their help and tested their patience. SH would like to thank Carolyn Hemsley for being a sounding board, supporter and proofreader. RP would like to thank our overseas colleagues for their input. The world community of burn injury specialists is small, but close knit, and we are always seeking better care for our patients throughout their lives. RP would also like to thank Shehan Hettiaratchy who has been the powerhouse behind this series. Without his enthusiasm and dogged determination to complete each stage this book and series would never have been published.

Finally, without feedback this ABC cannot improve. We value all your comments, both positive and negative; please send them in.

SH, RP, PD
2004

1   Introduction

Shehan Hettiaratchy, Peter Dziewulski

Burns are one of the most devastating conditions encountered in medicine. The injury represents an assault on all aspects of the patient, from the physical to the psychological. It affects all ages, from babies to elderly people, and is a problem in both the developed and developing world. All of us have experienced the severe pain that even a small burn can bring. However the pain and distress caused by a large burn are not limited to the immediate event. The visible physical and the invisible psychological scars are long lasting and often lead to chronic disability. Burn injuries represent a diverse and varied challenge to medical and paramedical staff. Correct management requires a skilled multidisciplinary approach that addresses all the problems facing a burn patient.

This series provides an overview of the most important aspects of burn injuries for hospital and non-hospital healthcare workers.

How common are burns?

In the United Kingdom about 250 000 people are burnt each year. Of these, 175 000 attend accident and emergency departments, and 13 000 of these are admitted to hospital. Some 1000 patients have severe enough burns to warrant formal fluid resuscitation; half of these are children aged under 12 years. In an average year 300 burn deaths occur. These UK figures are representative of most of the developed world countries, although some, such as the United States, have a higher incidence.

Burns are also a major problem in the developing world. Over two million burn injuries are thought to occur each year in India (population 500 million), but this may be a substantial underestimate. Mortality in the developing world is much higher than in the developed world. For example, Nepal has about 1700 burn deaths a year for a population of 20 million, giving a death rate 17 times that of Britain.

What are the causes of burns?

Most burns are due to flame injuries. Burns due to scalds are the next most common. The most infrequent burns are those caused by electrocution and chemical injuries. The type of burns suffered is related to the type of patient injured. It is therefore useful to break down burn aetiology by patient groups as this reveals the varying causes of injury. In most groups there is a male predominance. The only exception is in elderly people, among whom more women are injured because of the preponderance of women in that population.

Who gets burnt?

Young children—Children aged up to 4 years comprise 20% of all patients with burn injuries. Most injuries (70%) are scalds due to children spilling hot liquids or being exposed to hot bathing water. These mechanisms can lead to large area burns. Because of changes in the design and material of night clothing, flame burns are less common than they were. Boys are more likely to be injured, a reflection of the behavioural differences between boys and girls.

Older children and adolescents—10% of burns happen to children between the ages of 5 and 14. Teenagers are often

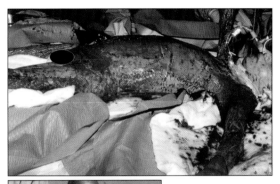

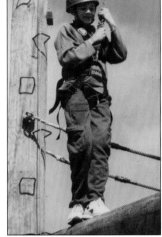

Top: Child with 70% full thickness burns, which required resuscitation, intensive care support, and extensive debridement and skin grafting. Left: The same child one year later at a burns camp, having made a good recovery. A reasonable outcome is possible even with severe burn injuries

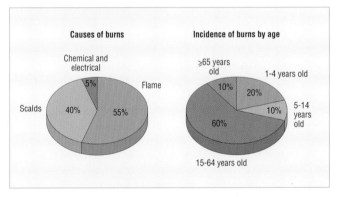

Causes of burns (left) and incidence of burns by age (right)

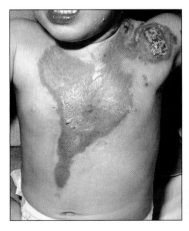

Scald in young child caused by spilling hot liquid. Most of the burn is superficial, except for the patch on the shoulder, which required a skin graft and which healed well

injured from illicit activities involving accelerants, such as petrol, or electrocution.

Working age—Most burns (>60%) occur in patients aged 15-64. These are mainly due to flame burns, and up to a third are due to work related incidents.

Elderly people—Some 10% of burns occur in people aged over 65. Various effects of ageing (such as immobility, slowed reactions, and decreased dexterity) mean elderly people are at risk from scalds, contact burns, and flame burns.

Compromising factors—Burn victims' health is often compromised by some other factor, such as alcoholism, epilepsy, or chronic psychiatric or medical illness. All such problems need to be addressed when managing patients in order to speed recovery and prevent repetition of injury.

Care of a major burn injury

The main aims of burn care are to restore form, function, and feeling, and burn management can be divided up into seven phases—rescue, resuscitate, retrieve, resurface, rehabilitate, reconstruct, and review.

Rescue—The aim is to get the individual away from the source of the injury and provide first aid. This is often done by non-professionals—friends, relatives, bystanders, etc.

Resuscitate—Immediate support must be provided for any failing organ system. This usually involves administering fluid to maintain the circulatory system but may also involve supporting the cardiac, renal, and respiratory systems.

Retrieve—After initial evacuation to an accident and emergency department, patients with serious burns may need transfer to a specialist burns unit for further care.

Resurface—The skin and tissues that have been damaged by the burn must be repaired. This can be achieved by various means, from simple dressings to aggressive surgical debridement and skin grafting.

Rehabilitate—This begins on the day a patient enters hospital and continues for years after he or she has left. The aim is to return patients, as far as is possible, to their pre-injury level of physical, emotional, and psychological wellbeing.

Reconstruct—The scarring that results from burns often leads to functional impairment that must be addressed. The operations needed to do this are often complex and may need repeating as a patient grows or the scars re-form.

Review—Burn patients, especially children, require regular review for many years so that problems can be identified early and solutions provided.

The complexity of the injury and the chronic nature of the sequelae of burns require an integrated multidisciplinary approach with long follow up. Only such management can lead to the best outcomes for burn patients.

Prognostication in major burns

Determining whether someone will survive a severe burn injury is not simple but is important. Aggressive treatment for someone with a non-survivable injury is inhumane, and it is inappropriate not to treat a patient who has a severe but potentially survivable injury. Unfortunately, there is no exact way to predict who will survive a burn injury. Several formulae have been devised to estimate the risk of death after burn injury. None has been evaluated prospectively in large trials, however, and so they should be used only for audit purposes. It is also inappropriate to apply generic formulae to individuals. Each patient should be considered individually.

Certain factors increase the risk of death. The most important are increasing age, increasing burn size, and the

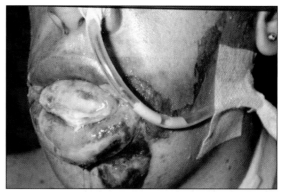
Burn incurred by an adolescent boy while inhaling butane gas. There was full thickness damage to the lower lip, which required debridement and extensive reconstruction

---

Aims of burn care

Restore form—Return the damaged area to as close to normality as is possible

Restore function—Maximise patient's ability to perform pre-injury activities

Restore feeling—Enable psychological and emotional recovery

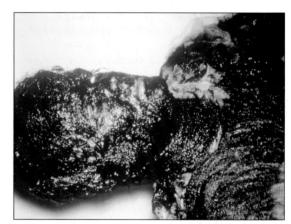
Bitumen burns to face in work related incident

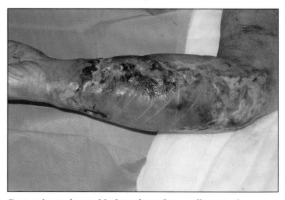
Contact burns in an elderly patient after a collapse and prolonged contact with a radiator. Treatment required excision and split skin grafting as well as investigation into the cause of the collapse

presence of an inhalational injury. Exactly how these factors interrelate is not clear. Evidence suggests that a patient aged over 60 with a burn covering more than 40% of body surface area and an inhalational injury has a >90% chance of dying.

As well as assessing the injury, it is also important to make some estimation of the patient's quality of life before the burn. This can be obtained from relatives, carers, or the patient. Deciding not to resuscitate a patient is difficult. It is often useful to get a consensus opinion from the whole burn team.

Burn prevention and fire safety

The fact that 90% of burn injuries are preventable has led to many attempts to decrease their incidence. These attempts fall into two main categories—education and legislation. Education is an "active" process that requires a change in an individual's behaviour. Legislation is "passive" and is independent of a person's actions. Both have advantages and disadvantages.

Education—The most successful campaigns have targeted specific burn aetiologies or populations. A good example of this is the campaign to reduce chip pan fires in Britain during the late 1970s. This led to a 30% reduction in the incidence of burns due to chip pan fires. The main problem with educational prevention is that it relies on changing the way individuals behave. This means the message must be repeated regularly, as shown by the UK government launching a second chip pan fire campaign in 1999. However, a successful educational campaign has an instantaneous and widespread impact.

Legislation—Legislation (such as the compulsory fitting of sprinklers in commercial buildings) has led to substantial decreases in burn injury. The main problem with legislation is that it takes time to pass and to have an effect. Compliance must also be obtained and maintained. However, as it does not rely on a change in individuals' actions, legislation can be effective.

Effective prevention requires both passive and active elements. The basis for all prevention is good epidemiological data to reveal specific causes of burns and at risk populations, both of which can be targeted. The UK government is currently running the "Fire kills" campaign, which covers all aspects of domestic fire prevention and safety. The related website, www.firekills.gov.uk, is an excellent source of information.

Some risk factors for burns are not easy to change. Overcrowding, poor housing, and the other attributes of poverty are major contributors to the risk of burn injuries.

Competing interests: RP has been reimbursed by Johnson & Johnson, manufacturer of Integra, and Smith & Nephew, manufacturer of Acticoat and TransCyte, for attending symposiums on burn care.

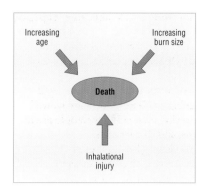

Factors that increase the risk of death after a major burn

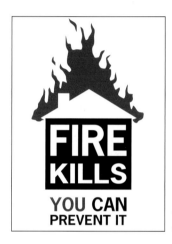

UK government's "Fire kills" campaign started in 2002

Information in UK government's "Fire kills" campaign

"Top 10 safety tips"

How to make your house a safe home
- Fit a smoke alarm and check it regularly
- Make a fire action plan so that everyone in your house knows how to escape in the event of fire
- Take care when cooking with hot oil and think about using thermostatically controlled deep fat fryers
- Never leave lit candles unattended
- Ensure cigarettes are stubbed out and disposed of carefully
- Never smoke in bed
- Keep matches and lighters away from children
- Keep clothing away from heating appliances
- Take care in the kitchen. Accidents while cooking account for 59% of fires in the home
- Take special care when you are tired or when you've been drinking. Half of all deaths in domestic fires occur between 10 pm and 8 am

On finding a fire in the home
- Get out
- Stay out
- Call 999 (telephone number for UK emergency services)

Key points
- Burns are a major cause of injury and death worldwide
- Flame burns are the most common type
- Young children, elderly people, and those who are mentally or physically compromised are at particular risk
- Death is more likely with increasing age, increasing burn size, and presence of inhalational injury
- 90% of burns are preventable

Further reading
- Wilkinson E. The epidemiology of burns in secondary care, in a population of 2.6 million people. *Burns* 1998;24:139-43
- Ryan CM, Schoenfeld DA, Thorpe WP, Sheridan RL, Cassem EH, Tompkins RG. Objective estimates of the probability of death from burn injuries. *N Engl J Med* 1998;338:362-6
- Fire kills. You can prevent it. www.firekills.gov.uk
- Herndon D. *Total burn care.* 2nd ed. London: WB Saunders, 2002
- National Community Fire Safety Centre Toolbox. www.firesafetytoolbox.org.uk
- Liao C-C, Rossignol AM. Landmarks in burn prevention. *Burns* 2000;26:422-34

2 Pathophysiology and types of burns

Shehan Hettiaratchy, Peter Dziewulski

Understanding the pathophysiology of a burn injury is important for effective management. In addition, different causes lead to different injury patterns, which require different management. It is therefore important to understand how a burn was caused and what kind of physiological response it will induce.

The body's response to a burn

Burn injuries result in both local and systemic responses.

Local response
The three zones of a burn were described by Jackson in 1947.

Zone of coagulation—This occurs at the point of maximum damage. In this zone there is irreversible tissue loss due to coagulation of the constituent proteins.

Zone of stasis—The surrounding zone of stasis is characterised by decreased tissue perfusion. The tissue in this zone is potentially salvageable. The main aim of burns resuscitation is to increase tissue perfusion here and prevent any damage becoming irreversible. Additional insults—such as prolonged hypotension, infection, or oedema—can convert this zone into an area of complete tissue loss.

Zone of hyperaemia—In this outermost zone tissue perfusion is increased. The tissue here will invariably recover unless there is severe sepsis or prolonged hypoperfusion.

These three zones of a burn are three dimensional, and loss of tissue in the zone of stasis will lead to the wound deepening as well as widening.

Systemic response
The release of cytokines and other inflammatory mediators at the site of injury has a systemic effect once the burn reaches 30% of total body surface area.

Cardiovascular changes—Capillary permeability is increased, leading to loss of intravascular proteins and fluids into the interstitial compartment. Peripheral and splanchnic vasoconstriction occurs. Myocardial contractility is decreased, possibly due to release of tumour necrosis factor α. These changes, coupled with fluid loss from the burn wound, result in systemic hypotension and end organ hypoperfusion.

Respiratory changes—Inflammatory mediators cause bronchoconstriction, and in severe burns adult respiratory distress syndrome can occur.

Metabolic changes—The basal metabolic rate increases up to three times its original rate. This, coupled with splanchnic hypoperfusion, necessitates early and aggressive enteral feeding to decrease catabolism and maintain gut integrity.

Immunological changes—Non-specific down regulation of the immune response occurs, affecting both cell mediated and humoral pathways.

Mechanisms of injury

Thermal injuries
Scalds—About 70% of burns in children are caused by scalds. They also often occur in elderly people. The common mechanisms are spilling hot drinks or liquids or being exposed

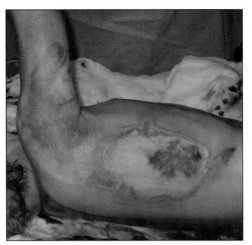

Clinical image of burn zones. There is central necrosis, surrounded by the zones of stasis and of hyperaemia

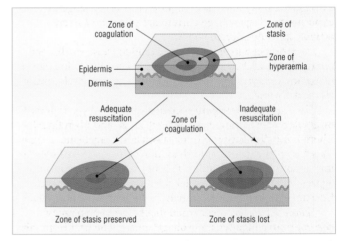

Jackson's burns zones and the effects of adequate and inadequate resuscitation

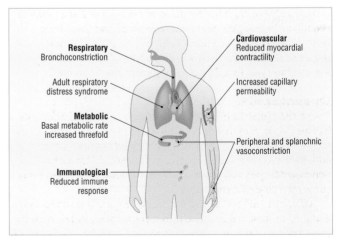

Systemic changes that occur after a burn injury

to hot bathing water. Scalds tend to cause superficial to superficial dermal burns (see later for burn depth).

Flame—Flame burns comprise 50% of adult burns. They are often associated with inhalational injury and other concomitant trauma. Flame burns tend to be deep dermal or full thickness.

Contact—In order to get a burn from direct contact, the object touched must either have been extremely hot or the contact was abnormally long. The latter is a more common reason, and these types of burns are commonly seen in people with epilepsy or those who misuse alcohol or drugs. They are also seen in elderly people after a loss of consciousness; such a presentation requires a full investigation as to the cause of the blackout. Burns from brief contact with very hot substances are usually due to industrial accidents. Contact burns tend to be deep dermal or full thickness.

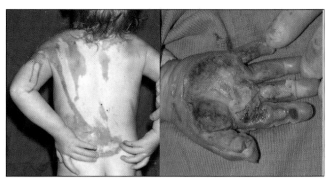

Examples of a scald burn (left) and a contact burn from a hot iron (right) in young children

Electrical injuries

Some 3-4% of burn unit admissions are caused by electrical injuries. An electric current will travel through the body from one point to another, creating "entry" and "exit" points. The tissue between these two points can be damaged by the current. The amount of heat generated, and hence the level of tissue damage, is equal to $0.24 \times (\text{voltage})^2 \times \text{resistance}$. The voltage is therefore the main determinant of the degree of tissue damage, and it is logical to divide electrical injuries into those caused by low voltage, domestic current and those due to high voltage currents. High voltage injuries can be further divided into "true" high tension injuries, caused by high voltage current passing through the body, and "flash" injuries, caused by tangential exposure to a high voltage current arc where no current actually flows through the body.

Domestic electricity—Low voltages tend to cause small, deep contact burns at the exit and entry sites. The alternating nature of domestic current can interfere with the cardiac cycle, giving rise to arrhythmias.

"True" high tension injuries occur when the voltage is 1000 V or greater. There is extensive tissue damage and often limb loss. There is usually a large amount of soft and bony tissue necrosis. Muscle damage gives rise to rhabdomyolysis, and renal failure may occur with these injuries. This injury pattern needs more aggressive resuscitation and debridement than other burns. Contact with voltage greater than 70 000 V is invariably fatal.

"Flash" injury can occur when there has been an arc of current from a high tension voltage source. The heat from this arc can cause superficial flash burns to exposed body parts, typically the face and hands. However, clothing can also be set alight, giving rise to deeper burns. No current actually passes through the victim's body.

A particular concern after an electrical injury is the need for cardiac monitoring. There is good evidence that if the patient's electrocardiogram on admission is normal and there is no history of loss of consciousness, then cardiac monitoring is not required. If there are electrocardiographic abnormalities or a loss of consciousness, 24 hours of monitoring is advised.

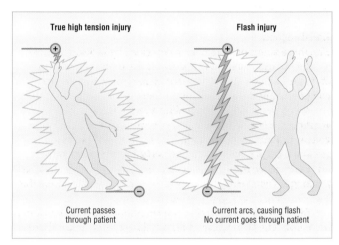

Differences between true high tension burn and flash burn

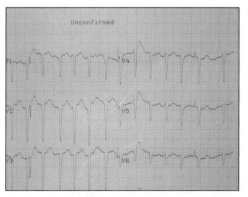

Electrocardiogram after electrocution showing atrial fibrillation

Chemical injuries

Chemical injuries are usually as a result of industrial accidents but may occur with household chemical products. These burns tend to be deep, as the corrosive agent continues to cause coagulative necrosis until completely removed. Alkalis tend to penetrate deeper and cause worse burns than acids. Cement is a common cause of alkali burns.

Certain industrial agents may require specific treatments in addition to standard first aid. Hydrofluoric acid, widely used for glass etching and in the manufacture of circuit boards, is one of the more common culprits. It causes a continuing, penetrating

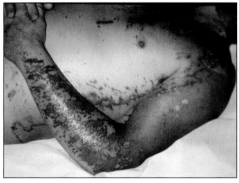

Chemical burn due to spillage of sulphuric acid

injury and must be neutralised with calcium gluconate, either applied topically in a gel or injected into the affected tissues.

The initial management of all chemical burns is the same irrespective of the agent. All contaminated clothing must be removed, and the area thoroughly irrigated. This is often best achieved by showering the patient. This has been shown to limit the depth of the burn. Litmus paper can be used to confirm removal of alkali or acid. Eye injuries should be irrigated copiously and referred to an ophthalmologist.

Non-accidental injury

An estimated 3-10% of paediatric burns are due to non-accidental injury. Detecting these injuries is important as up to 30% of children who are repeatedly abused die. Usually young children (<3 years old) are affected. As with other non-accidental injuries, the history and the pattern of injury may arouse suspicion. A social history is also important. Abuse is more common in poor households with single or young parents. Such abuse is not limited to children: elderly and other dependent adults are also at risk. A similar assessment can be made in these scenarios.

It is natural for non-accidental injury to trigger anger among healthcare workers. However, it is important that all members of the team remain non-confrontational and try to establish a relationship with the perpetrators. The time around the burn injury is an excellent opportunity to try to break the cycle of abuse. In addition, it is likely that the patient will eventually be discharged back into the care of the individuals who caused the injury. As well as treating the physical injury, the burn team must try to prevent further abuse by changing the relationship dynamics between victim and abuser(s).

Any suspicion of non-accidental injury should lead to immediate admission of the child to hospital, irrespective of how trivial the burn is, and the notification of social services. The team should carry out the following:
- Examine for other signs of abuse
- Photograph all injuries
- Obtain a team opinion about parent-child interaction
- Obtain other medical information (from general practitioner, health visitor, referring hospital)
- Interview family members separately about the incident (check for inconsistencies) and together (observe interaction).

It should be remembered that the injury does not have to be caused deliberately for social services to intervene; inadequate supervision of children mandates their involvement.

Specific chemical burns and treatments

Chromic acid—Rinse with dilute sodium hyposulphite
Dichromate salts—Rinse with dilute sodium hyposulphite
Hydrofluoric acid—10% calcium gluconate applied topically as a gel or injected

Injury pattern of non-accidental burns

- Obvious pattern from cigarettes, lighters, irons
- Burns to soles, palms, genitalia, buttocks, perineum
- Symmetrical burns of uniform depth
- No splash marks in a scald injury. A child falling into a bath will splash; one that is placed into it may not
- Restraint injuries on upper limbs
- Is there sparing of flexion creases—that is, was child in fetal position (position of protection) when burnt? Does this correlate to a "tide line" of scald—that is, if child is put into a fetal position, do the burns line up?
- Other signs of physical abuse—bruises of varied age, poorly kempt, lack of compliance with health care (such as no immunisations)

History of non-accidental burns

- Evasive or changing history
- Delayed presentation
- No explanation or an implausible mechanism given for the burn
- Inconsistency between age of the burn and age given by the history
- Inadequate supervision, such as child left in the care of inappropriate person (older sibling)
- Lack of guilt about the incident
- Lack of concern about treatment or prognosis

Further reading

- Kao CC, Garner WL. Acute burns. *Plast Reconstr Surg* 2000;105: 2482-93
- Andronicus M, Oates RK, Peat J, Spalding S, Martin H. Non-accidental burns in children. *Burns* 1998;24:552-8
- Herndon D. *Total burn care.* 2nd ed. London: WB Saunders, 2002
- Luce EA. Electrical burns. *Clin Plast Surg* 2000;27:133-43
- Kirkpatrick JJR, Enion DS, Burd DAR. Hydrofluoric acid burns; a review. *Burns* 1995;21:483-93
- Burnsurgery.org. www.burnsurgery.org

Key points

- A burn results in three distinct zones—coagulation, stasis, and hyperaemia
- The aim of burns resuscitation is to maintain perfusion of the zone of stasis
- Systemic response occurs once a burn is greater than 30% of total body surface area
- Different burn mechanisms lead to different injury patterns
- Identification of non-accidental burn injury is important

3 First aid and treatment of minor burns

Jackie Hudspith, Sukh Rayatt

Some 250 000 burns occur annually in the United Kingdom. About 90% of these are minor and can be safely managed in primary care. Most of these will heal regardless of treatment, but the initial care can have a considerable influence on the cosmetic outcome. All burns should be assessed by taking an adequate history and examination.

First aid

The aims of first aid should be to stop the burning process, cool the burn, provide pain relief, and cover the burn.

Stop the burning process—The heat source should be removed. Flames should be doused with water or smothered with a blanket or by rolling the victim on the ground. Rescuers should take care to avoid burn injury to themselves. Clothing can retain heat, even in a scald burn, and should be removed as soon as possible. Adherent material, such as nylon clothing, should be left on. Tar burns should be cooled with water, but the tar itself should not be removed. In the case of electrical burns the victim should be disconnected from the source of electricity before first aid is attempted.

Cooling the burn—Active cooling removes heat and prevents progression of the burn. This is effective if performed within 20 minutes of the injury. Immersion or irrigation with running tepid water (15°C) should be continued for up to 20 minutes. This also removes noxious agents and reduces pain, and may reduce oedema by stabilising mast cells and histamine release. Iced water should not be used as intense vasoconstriction can cause burn progression. Cooling large areas of skin can lead to hypothermia, especially in children. Chemical burns should be irrigated with copious amounts of water.

Analgesia—Exposed nerve endings will cause pain. Cooling and simply covering the exposed burn will reduce the pain. Opioids may be required initially to control pain, but once first aid measures have been effective non-steroidal anti-inflammatory drugs such as ibuprofen or co-dydramol taken orally will suffice.

Covering the burn—Dressings should cover the burn area and keep the patient warm. Polyvinyl chloride film (cling film) is an ideal first aid cover. The commercially available roll is essentially sterile as long as the first few centimetres are discarded. This dressing is pliable, non-adherent, impermeable, acts as a barrier, and is transparent for inspection. It is important to lay this on the wound rather than wrapping the burn. This is especially important on limbs, as later swelling may lead to constriction. A blanket laid over the top will keep the patient warm. If cling film is not available then any clean cotton sheet (preferably sterile) can be used. Hand burns can be covered with a clear plastic bag so as not to restrict mobility. Avoid using wet dressings, as heat loss during transfer to hospital can be considerable.

Use of topical creams should be avoided at this stage as these may interfere with subsequent assessment of the burn. Cooling gels such as Burnshield are often used by paramedics. These are useful in cooling the burn and relieving pain in the initial stages.

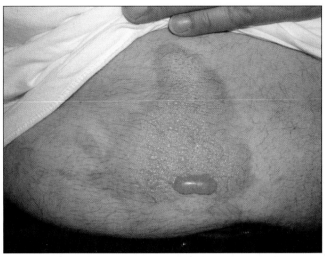
A superficial scald suitable for management in primary care

Benefits of cooling burn injuries with water

- Stops burning process
- Reduces pain
- Minimises oedema
- Cleanses wound

Cling film for dressing burn wounds

- Essentially sterile
- Lay on wound—Do not wrap around
- Non-adherent
- Pliable
- Transparent for inspection

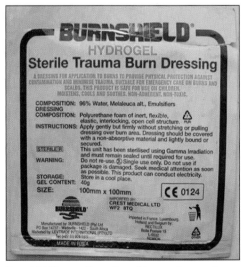
Burnshield is a cooling gel used to cover burn and reduce pain

Management of minor burns

The cause of injury and depth and extent of burn should be assessed in the same way as for more major burns and recorded. Similarly, associated illness or injuries must be considered (such as small burns as a result of fits, faints, or falls). Burns suitable for outpatient management are usually small and superficial and not affecting critical areas. Home circumstances should be considered, as even small injuries to the feet will progress if the legs are not elevated for at least 48 hours; this is rarely possible at home. Always consult a burns unit if in doubt about management

Once the decision has been taken to treat a burn patient as an outpatient, analgesia should be given and the wound thoroughly cleaned and a dressing applied (except on the face). Ensure that a follow up appointment is made.

There are a vast range of acceptable options in the outpatient management of minor burns. The following should be used as a guide

Cleaning the burn

It is important to realise that a new burn is essentially sterile, and every attempt should be made to keep it so. The burn wound should be thoroughly cleaned with soap and water or mild antibacterial wash such as dilute chlorohexidine. Routine use of antibiotics should be discouraged. There is some controversy over management of blisters, but large ones should probably be de-roofed, and dead skin removed with sterile scissors or a hypodermic needle. Smaller blisters should be left intact.

Dressings

Many different dressings are in use, with little or no data to support any individual approach. We favour covering the clean burn with a simple gauze dressing impregnated with paraffin (Jelonet). Avoid using topical creams as these will interfere with subsequent assessment of the burn. Apply a gauze pad over the dressing, followed by several layers of absorbent cotton wool. A firm crepe bandage applied in a figure of eight manner and secured with plenty of adhesive tape (Elastoplast) will prevent slippage of the dressing and shearing of the wound.

An elastic net dressing (Netelast) is useful for securing awkward areas such as the head and neck and chest. Limb burns should be elevated for the duration of treatment.

Dressing changes

The practice of subsequent dressing changes is varied. Ideally the dressing should be checked at 24 hours. The burn wound itself should be reassessed at 48 hours and the dressings changed, as they are likely to be soaked through. At this stage the depth of burn should be apparent, and topical agents such as Flamazine can be used.

Depending on how healing is progressing, dressing changes thereafter should be every three to five days. If the Jelonet dressing has become adherent, it should be left in place to avoid damage to delicate healing epithelium. If Flamazine is used it should be changed on alternate days. The dressing should be changed immediately if the wound becomes painful or smelly or the dressing becomes soaked ("strike through").

Any burn that has not healed within two weeks should be seen by a burn surgeon.

Specialist dressings

Many specialist dressings are available, some developed for specific cases, but most designed for their ease of use. The following are among the more widely used.

Minor burns suitable for outpatient management

- Partial thickness burns covering < 10% of total body surface area in adults
- Partial thickness burns covering < 5% of body surface area in children
- Full thickness burns covering < 1% of body surface
- No comorbidity

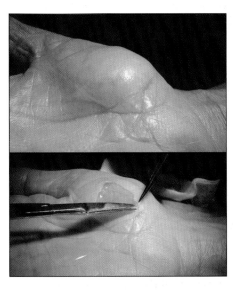

Large blister on thenar eminence restricting movement of hand (top). Blister is de-roofed using aseptic technique (bottom)

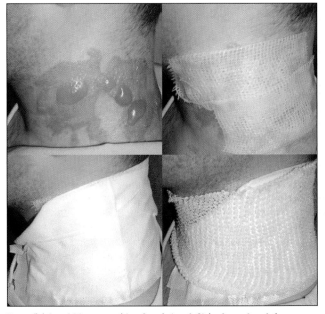

Superficial scald burn on side of neck (top left) is cleaned and then a layer of Jelonet applied over it (top right). Gauze square dressings on top of the Jelonet (bottom left) are held in place with a Netelast type of dressing (bottom right)

Dressing changes for burns

- Use aseptic technique
- First change after 48 hours, and every 3-5 days thereafter
- Criteria for early dressing change:
  Excessive "strike through" of fluid from wound
  Smelly wound
  Contaminated or soiled dressings
  Slipped dressings
  Signs of infection (such as fever)

Flamazine is silver sulfadiazine cream and is applied topically on the burn wound. It is effective against gram negative bacteria including *Pseudomonas*. Infection with the latter will cause the dressing to turn green with a distinctive smell. Apply the cream in a 3-5 mm thick layer and cover with gauze. It should be removed and reapplied every two days. There is a reported 3-5% incidence of reversible leucopenia.

Granulflex is a hydrocolloid dressing with a thin polyurethane foam sheet bonded onto a semipermeable film. The dressing is adhesive and waterproof and is therefore useful in awkward areas or where normal dressings are not suitable. It should be applied with a 2 cm border. By maintaining a moist atmosphere over the wound, it creates an environment suitable for healing. It usually needs to be changed every three or four days, but it can be left for seven days. A thinner version (Duoderm) is also available.

Mepitel is a flexible polyamide net coated with soft silicone to give a Jelonet-type of dressing that is non adhesive. It is a useful but expensive alternative to Jelonet when easy removal is desirable, such as with children.

Facial burns

Facial burns should be referred to a specialist unit. However, simple sunburn should be left exposed as dressings can be awkward to retain on the face. The wound should be cleansed twice daily with mild diluted chlorhexidine solution. The burn should be covered with a bland ointment such as liquid paraffin. This should be applied every 1-4 hours as necessary to minimise crust formation. Men should shave daily to reduce risk of infection. All patients should be advised to sleep propped up on two pillows for the first 48 hours to minimise facial oedema.

Follow up

Burns that fail to heal within three weeks should be referred to a plastic surgery unit for review. Healed burns will be sensitive and have dry scaly skin, which may develop pigmental changes. Daily application of moisturiser cream should be encouraged. Healed areas should be protected from the sun with sun block for 6-12 months. Pruritis is a common problem.

Physiotherapy—Patients with minor burns of limbs may need physiotherapy. It is important to identify these patients early and start therapy. Hypertrophic scars may benefit from scar therapy such as pressure garments or silicone. For these reasons, all healed burns should be reviewed at two months for referral to an occupational therapist if necessary.

Support and reassurance—Patients with burn injuries often worry about disfigurement and ugliness, at least in the short term, and parents of burnt children often have feelings of guilt. It is important to address these issues with reassurance.

Flamazine
- Silver sulfadiazine cream
- Covers gram negative bacteria including *Pseudomonas*
- Needs to be changed every 24-48 hours
- Makes burn seem white and should be avoided if burn needs reassessment

Management of facial burns
- Clean face twice a day with dilute chlorhexidine solution
- Cover with cream such as liquid paraffin on hourly basis
- Men should shave daily
- Sleep propped up on two pillows to minimise oedema

Pruritis
- Common in healing and healed burn wounds
- Aggravated by heat, stress, and physical activity
- Worst after healing
- Massage with aqueous cream or aloe vera cream
- Use antihistamines (such as chlorphenamine) and analgesics

Key points
- Initial first aid can influence final cosmetic outcome
- Cooling with tepid tap water is one of the most important first aid measures
- Routine use of antibiotics should be discouraged
- Simple dressings suffice
- Aseptic technique should be used for dressing changes
- If in doubt, seek advice from regional burns unit or plastic surgery department

Further reading
- Wilson G, French G. Plasticized polyvinylchloride as a temporary dressing for burns. *BMJ* 1987;294:556-7
- Davies JWL. Prompt cooling of the burned area: a review of benefits and the effector mechanisms. *Burns* 1982;9:1-6
- Slater RM, Hughes NC. A simplified method of treating burns of the hands. *Br J Plast Surg* 1971;24:296-300
- Herndon D. *Total burn care.* 2nd ed. London: Harcourt, 2002
- Settle J, ed. *Principles and practice of burns management.* Edinburgh: Churchill Livingstone, 1996
- National Burn Care Review. National burn injury referral guidelines. In: *Standards and strategy for burn care.* London: NBCR, 2001: 68-9

4 Initial management of a major burn: I—overview

Shehan Hettiaratchy, Remo Papini

A major burn is defined as a burn covering 25% or more of total body surface area, but any injury over more than 10% should be treated similarly. Rapid assessment is vital. The general approach to a major burn can be extrapolated to managing any burn. The most important points are to take an accurate history and make a detailed examination of the patient and the burn, to ensure that key information is not missed.

This article outlines the structure of the initial assessment. The next article will cover the detailed assessment of burn surface area and depth and how to calculate the fluid resuscitation formula.

History taking

The history of a burn injury can give valuable information about the nature and extent of the burn, the likelihood of inhalational injury, the depth of burn, and probability of other injuries. The exact mechanism of injury and any prehospital treatment must be established.

A patient's history must be obtained on admission, as this may be the only time that a first hand history is obtainable. Swelling may develop around the airway in the hours after injury and require intubation, making it impossible for the patient to give a verbal history. A brief medical history should be taken, outlining previous medical problems, medications, allergies, and vaccinations. Patients' smoking habits should be determined as these may affect blood gas analyses.

Primary survey

The initial management of a severely burnt patient is similar to that of any trauma patient. A modified "advanced trauma life support" primary survey is performed, with particular emphasis on assessment of the airway and breathing. The burn injury must not distract from this sequential assessment, otherwise serious associated injuries may be missed.

A—Airway with cervical spine control

An assessment must be made as to whether the airway is compromised or is at risk of compromise. The cervical spine should be protected unless it is definitely not injured. Inhalation of hot gases will result in a burn above the vocal cords. This burn will become oedematous over the following hours, especially after fluid resuscitation has begun. This means that an airway that is patent on arrival at hospital may occlude after admission. This can be a particular problem in small children.

Direct inspection of the oropharynx should be done by a senior anaesthetist. If there is any concern about the patency of the airway then intubation is the safest policy. However, an unnecessary intubation and sedation could worsen a patient's condition, so the decision to intubate should be made carefully.

B—Breathing

All burn patients should receive 100% oxygen through a humidified non-rebreathing mask on presentation. Breathing problems are considered to be those that affect the respiratory system below the vocal cords. There are several ways that a burn injury can compromise respiration.

Initial assessment of a major burn
- Perform an ABCDEF primary survey
  A—Airway with cervical spine control, B—Breathing, C—Circulation, D—Neurological disability, E—Exposure with environmental control, F—Fluid resuscitation
- Assess burn size and depth (see later article for detail)
- Establish good intravenous access and give fluids
- Give analgesia
- Catheterise patient or establish fluid balance monitoring
- Take baseline blood samples for investigation
- Dress wound
- Perform secondary survey, reassess, and exclude or treat associated injuries
- Arrange safe transfer to specialist burns facility

Key points of a burn history

Exact mechanism
- Type of burn agent (scald, flame, electrical, chemical)
- How did it come into contact with patient?
- What first aid was performed?
- What treatment has been started?
- Is there risk of concomitant injuries (such as fall from height, road traffic crash, explosion)?
- Is there risk of inhalational injuries (did burn occur in an enclosed space)?

Exact timings
- When did the injury occur?
- How long was patient exposed to energy source?
- How long was cooling applied?
- When was fluid resuscitation started?

Exact injury
Scalds
- What was the liquid? Was it boiling or recently boiled?
- If tea or coffee, was milk in it?
- Was a solute in the liquid? (Raises boiling temperature and causes worse injury, such as boiling rice)

Electrical injuries
- What was the voltage (domestic or industrial)?
- Was there a flash or arcing?
- Contact time

Chemical injuries
- What was the chemical?

Is there any suspicion of non-accidental injury?
- See previous article

Airway management

Signs of inhalational injury
- History of flame burns or burns in an enclosed space
- Full thickness or deep dermal burns to face, neck, or upper torso
- Singed nasal hair
- Carbonaceous sputum or carbon particles in oropharynx

Indications for intubation
- Erythema or swelling of oropharynx on direct visualisation
- Change in voice, with hoarseness or harsh cough
- Stridor, tachypnoea, or dyspnoea

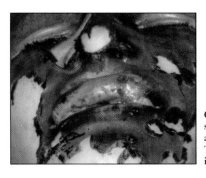

Carbonaceous particles staining a patient's face after a burn in an enclosed space. This suggests there is inhalational injury

Mechanical restriction of breathing—Deep dermal or full thickness circumferential burns of the chest can limit chest excursion and prevent adequate ventilation. This may require escharotomies (see next article).

Blast injury—If there has been an explosion, blast lung can complicate ventilation. Penetrating injuries can cause tension pneumothoraces, and the blast itself can cause lung contusions and alveolar trauma and lead to adult respiratory distress syndrome.

Smoke inhalation—The products of combustion, though cooled by the time they reach the lungs, act as direct irritants to the lungs, leading to bronchospasm, inflammation, and bronchorrhoea. The ciliary action of pneumocytes is impaired, exacerbating the situation. The inflammatory exudate created is not cleared, and atelectasis or pneumonia follows. The situation can be particularly severe in asthmatic patients. Non-invasive management can be attempted, with nebulisers and positive pressure ventilation with some positive end-expiratory pressure. However, patients may need a period of ventilation, as this allows adequate oxygenation and permits regular lung toileting.

Carboxyhaemoglobin—Carbon monoxide binds to deoxyhaemoglobin with 40 times the affinity of oxygen. It also binds to intracellular proteins, particularly the cytochrome oxidase pathway. These two effects lead to intracellular and extracellular hypoxia. Pulse oximetry cannot differentiate between oxyhaemoglobin and carboxyhaemoglobin, and may therefore give normal results. However, blood gas analysis will reveal metabolic acidosis and raised carboxyhaemoglobin levels but may not show hypoxia. Treatment is with 100% oxygen, which displaces carbon monoxide from bound proteins six times faster than does atmospheric oxygen. Patients with carboxyhaemoglobin levels greater than 25-30% should be ventilated. Hyperbaric therapy is rarely practical and has not been proved to be advantageous. It takes longer to shift the carbon monoxide from the cytochrome oxidase pathway than from haemoglobin, so oxygen therapy should be continued until the metabolic acidosis has cleared.

C—Circulation

Intravenous access should be established with two large bore cannulas preferably placed through unburnt tissue. This is an opportunity to take blood for checking full blood count, urea and electrolytes, blood group, and clotting screen. Peripheral circulation must be checked. Any deep or full thickness circumferential extremity burn can act as a tourniquet, especially once oedema develops after fluid resuscitation. This may not occur until some hours after the burn. If there is any suspicion of decreased perfusion due to circumferential burn, the tissue must be released with escharotomies (see next article).

Profound hypovolaemia is not the normal initial response to a burn. If a patient is hypotensive then it is may be due to delayed presentation, cardiogenic dysfunction, or an occult source of blood loss (chest, abdomen, or pelvis).

D—Neurological disability

All patients should be assessed for responsiveness with the Glasgow coma scale; they may be confused because of hypoxia or hypovolaemia.

E—Exposure with environment control

The whole of a patient should be examined (including the back) to get an accurate estimate of the burn area (see later) and to check for any concomitant injuries. Burn patients, especially children, easily become hypothermic. This will lead to hypoperfusion and deepening of burn wounds. Patients should be covered and warmed as soon as possible.

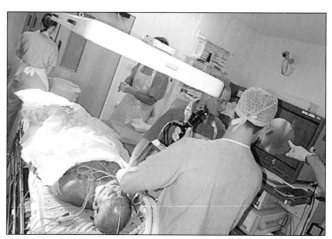

Acute bronchoscopy being performed to assess amount of damage to the bronchial tree. Patient has been covered in a blanket and a heat lamp placed overhead to prevent excessive cooling

Signs of carboxyhaemoglobinaemia

COHb levels	Symptoms
0-10%	Minimal (normal level in heavy smokers)
10-20%	Nausea, headache
20-30%	Drowsiness, lethargy
30-40%	Confusion, agitation
40-50%	Coma, respiratory depression
>50%	Death

COHb = Carboxyhaemoglobin

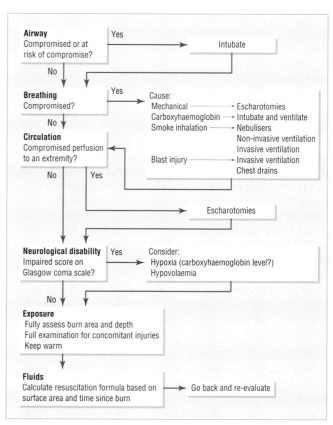

Algorithm for primary survey of a major burn injury

F—Fluid resuscitation

The resuscitation regimen should be determined and begun. This is based on the estimation of the burn area, and the detailed calculation is covered in the next article. A urinary catheter is mandatory in all adults with injuries covering >20% of total body surface area to monitor urine output. Children's urine output can be monitored with external catchment devices or by weighing nappies provided the injury is <20% of total body area. In children the interosseous route can be used for fluid administration if intravenous access cannot be obtained, but should be replaced by intravenous lines as soon as possible.

Analgesia

Superficial burns can be extremely painful. All patients with large burns should receive intravenous morphine at a dose appropriate to body weight. This can be easily titrated against pain and respiratory depression. The need for further doses should be assessed within 30 minutes.

Investigations

The amount of investigations will vary with the type of burn.

Secondary survey

At the end of the primary survey and the start of emergency management, a secondary survey should be performed. This is a head to toe examination to look for any concomitant injuries.

Dressing the wound

Once the surface area and depth of a burn have been estimated, the burn wound should be washed and any loose skin removed. Blisters should be deroofed for ease of dressing, except for palmar blisters (painful), unless these are large enough to restrict movement. The burn should then be dressed.

For an acute burn which will be referred to a burn centre, cling film is an ideal dressing as it protects the wound, reduces heat and evaporative losses, and does not alter the wound appearance. This will permit accurate evaluation by the burn team later. Flamazine should not be used on a burn that is to be referred immediately, since it makes assessment of depth more difficult.

Referral to a burns unit

The National Burn Care Review has established referral guidelines to specialist units. Burns are divided into complex burns (those that require specialist intervention) and non-complex burns (those that do not require immediate admission to a specialist unit). Complex burns should be referred automatically. If you are not sure whether a burn should be referred, discuss the case with your local burns unit. It is also important to discuss all burns that are not healed within two weeks.

Competing interests: RP has been reimbursed by Johnson & Johnson, manufacturer of Integra, and Smith & Nephew, manufacturer of Acticoat and TransCyte, for attending symposia on burn care.

Investigations for major burns*

General
- Full blood count, packed cell volume, urea and electrolyte concentration, clotting screen
- Blood group, and save or crossmatch serum

Electrical injuries
- 12 lead electrocardiography
- Cardiac enzymes (for high tension injuries)

Inhalational injuries
- Chest x ray
- Arterial blood gas analysis
  Can be useful in any burn, as the base excess is predictive of the amount of fluid resuscitation required
  Helpful for determining success of fluid resuscitation and essential with inhalational injuries or exposure to carbon monoxide

*Any concomitant trauma will have its own investigations

Indications for referral to a burns unit

All complex injuries should be referred
A burn injury is more likely to be complex if associated with:
- Extremes of age—under 5 or over 60 years
- Site of injury
  Face, hands, or perineum
  Feet (dermal or full thickness loss)
  Any flexure, particularly the neck or axilla
  Circumferential dermal or full thickness burn of limb, torso, or neck
- Inhalational injury
  Any substantial injury, excluding pure carbon monoxide poisoning
- Mechanism of injury
  Chemical injury >5% of total body surface area
  Exposure to ionising radiation
  High pressure steam injury
  High tension electrical injury
  Hydrofluoric acid burn >1% of total body surface area
  Suspicion of non-accidental injury
- Large size (dermal or full thickness loss)
  Paediatric (<16 years old) >5% of total body surface area
  Adult (≥16 years) >10% of total body surface area
- Coexisting conditions
  Any serious medical conditions (cardiac dysfunction, immunosuppression, pregnancy)
  Any associated injuries (fractures, head injuries, crush injuries)

Key points
- Perform a systematic assessment as with any trauma patient (don't get distracted by the burn)
- Beware of airway compromise
- Provide adequate analgesia
- Exclude any concomitant injuries
- Discuss with a burns unit early
- If in doubt, reassess

Further reading
- Sheridan R. Burns. *Crit Care Med* 2002;30:S500-14
- British Burn Association. Emergency management of severe burns course manual, UK version. Wythenshawe Hospital, Manchester, 1996
- Herndon D. *Total burn care*. 2nd ed. London: WB Saunders, 2002
- Kao CC, Garner WL. Acute burns. *Plast Reconstr Surg* 2000;105: 2482-93
- Burnsurgery.org. www.burnsurgery.org

5 Initial management of a major burn: II—assessment and resuscitation

Shehan Hettiaratchy, Remo Papini

Assessment of burn area

Assessment of burn area tends to be done badly, even by those who are expert at it. There are three commonly used methods of estimating burn area, and each has a role in different scenarios. When calculating burn area, erythema should not be included. This may take a few hours to fade, so some overestimation is inevitable if the burn is estimated acutely.

Palmar surface—The surface area of a patient's palm (including fingers) is roughly 0.8% of total body surface area. Palmar surface are can be used to estimate relatively small burns (<15% of total surface area) or very large burns (>85%, when unburnt skin is counted). For medium sized burns, it is inaccurate.

Wallace rule of nines—This is a good, quick way of estimating medium to large burns in adults. The body is divided into areas of 9%, and the total burn area can be calculated. It is not accurate in children.

Lund and Browder chart—This chart, if used correctly, is the most accurate method. It compensates for the variation in body shape with age and therefore can give an accurate assessment of burns area in children.

It is important that all of the burn is exposed and assessed. During assessment, the environment should be kept warm, and small segments of skin exposed sequentially to reduce heat loss. Pigmented skin can be difficult to assess, and in such cases it may be necessary to remove all the loose epidermal layers to calculate burn size.

Resuscitation regimens

Fluid losses from the injury must be replaced to maintain homoeostasis. There is no ideal resuscitation regimen, and many are in use. All the fluid formulas are only guidelines, and their success relies on adjusting the amount of resuscitation fluid against monitored physiological parameters. The main aim of resuscitation is to maintain tissue perfusion to the zone of stasis and so prevent the burn deepening. This is not easy, as too little fluid will cause hypoperfusion whereas too much will lead to oedema that will cause tissue hypoxia.

The greatest amount of fluid loss in burn patients is in the first 24 hours after injury. For the first eight to 12 hours, there is a general shift of fluid from the intravascular to interstitial fluid compartments. This means that any fluid given during this time will rapidly leave the intravascular compartment. Colloids have no advantage over crystalloids in maintaining circulatory volume. Fast fluid boluses probably have little benefit, as a rapid rise in intravascular hydrostatic pressure will just drive more fluid out of the circulation. However, much protein is lost through the burn wound, so there is a need to replace this oncotic loss. Some resuscitation regimens introduce colloid after the first eight hours, when the loss of fluid from the intravascular space is decreasing.

Burns covering more than 15% of total body surface area in adults and more than 10% in children warrant formal resuscitation. Again these are guidelines, and experienced staff can exercise some discretion either way. The most commonly used resuscitation formula is the Parkland formula, a pure crystalloid formula. It has the advantage of being easy to

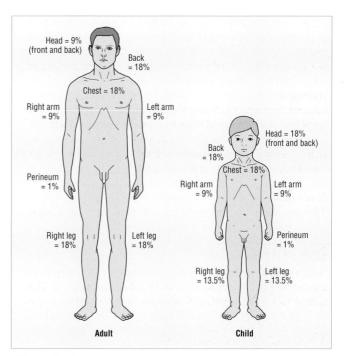

Wallace rule of nines

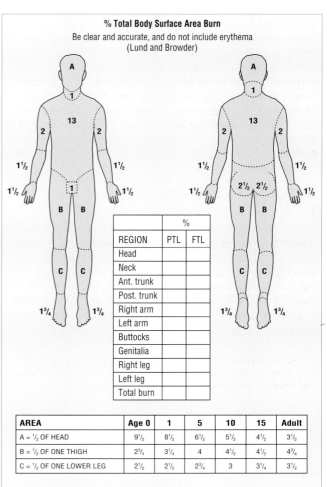

Lund and Browder chart

calculate and the rate is titrated against urine output. This calculates the amount of fluid required in the first 24 hours. Children require maintenance fluid in addition to this. The starting point for resuscitation is the time of injury, not the time of admission. Any fluid already given should be deducted from the calculated requirement.

At the end of 24 hours, colloid infusion is begun at a rate of 0.5 ml×(total burn surface area (%))×(body weight (kg)), and maintenance crystalloid (usually dextrose-saline) is continued at a rate of 1.5 ml×(burn area)×(body weight). The end point to aim for is a urine output of 0.5-1.0 ml/kg/hour in adults and 1.0-1.5 ml/kg/hour in children.

High tension electrical injuries require substantially more fluid (up to 9 ml×(burn area)×(body weight) in the first 24 hours) and a higher urine output (1.5-2 ml/kg/hour). Inhalational injuries also require more fluid.

In Britain Hartman's solution (sodium chloride 0.6%, sodium lactate 0.25%, potassium chloride 0.04%, calcium chloride 0.027%) is the most commonly used crystalloid. Colloid use is controversial: some units introduce colloid after eight hours, as the capillary leak begins to shut down, whereas others wait until 24 hours. Fresh frozen plasma is often used in children, and albumin or synthetic high molecular weight starches are used in adults.

The above regimens are merely guidelines to the probable amount of fluid required. This should be continuously adjusted according to urine output and other physiological parameters (pulse, blood pressure, and respiratory rate). Investigations at intervals of four to six hours are mandatory for monitoring a patient's resuscitation status. These include packed cell volume, plasma sodium, base excess, and lactate.

Burns units use different resuscitation formulas, and it is best to contact the local unit for advice.

Escharotomies

A circumferential deep dermal or full thickness burn is inelastic and on an extremity will not stretch. Fluid resuscitation leads to the development of burn wound oedema and swelling of the tissue beneath this inelastic burnt tissue. Tissue pressures rise and can impair peripheral circulation. Circumferential chest burns can also cause problems by limiting chest excursion and impairing ventilation. Both of these situations require escharotomy, division of the burn eschar. Only the burnt tissue is divided, not any underlying fascia, differentiating this procedure from a fasciotomy.

Incisions are made along the midlateral or medial aspects of the limbs, avoiding any underlying structures. For the chest, longitudinal incisions are made down each midaxillary line to the subcostal region. The lines are joined up by a chevron incision running parallel to the subcostal margin. This creates a mobile breastplate that moves with ventilation. Escharotomies are best done with electrocautery, as they tend to bleed. They are then packed with Kaltostat alginate dressing and dressed with the burn.

Although they are an urgent procedure, escharotomies are best done in an operating theatre by experienced staff. They should be discussed with the local burns unit, and performed under instruction only when transfer is delayed by several hours. Initially, at risk limbs should be elevated and observed.

Assessment of burn depth

The depth of burn is related to the amount of energy delivered in the injury and to the relative thickness of the skin (the dermis is thinner in very young and very old people).

Parkland formula for burns resuscitation

Total fluid requirement in 24 hours =
   4 ml×(total burn surface area (%))×(body weight (kg))
   50% given in first 8 hours
   50% given in next 16 hours
Children receive maintenance fluid in addition, at hourly rate of
   4 ml/kg for first 10 kg of body weight *plus*
   2 ml/kg for second 10 kg of body weight *plus*
   1 ml/kg for >20 kg of body weight

End point

Urine output of 0.5-1.0 ml/kg/hour in adults
Urine output of 1.0-1.5 ml/kg/hour in children

Worked examples of burns resuscitation

Fluid resuscitation regimen for an adult

A 25 year old man weighing 70 kg with a 30% flame burn was admitted at 4 pm. His burn occurred at 3 pm.

1) Total fluid requirement for first 24 hours
4 ml×(30% total burn surface area)×(70 kg) = 8400 ml in 24 hours

2) Half to be given in first 8 hours, half over the next 16 hours
Will receive 4200 ml during 0-8 hours and 4200 ml during 8-24 hours

3) Subtract any fluid already received from amount required for first 8 hours
Has already received 1000 ml from emergency services, and so needs further 3200 ml in first 8 hours after injury

4) Calculate hourly infusion rate for first 8 hours
Divide amount of fluid calculated in (3) by time left until it is 8 hours after burn
Burn occurred at 3 pm, so 8 hour point is 11 pm. It is now 4 pm, so need 3200 ml over next 7 hours:
   3200/7 = 457 ml/hour from 4 pm to 11 pm

5) Calculate hourly infusion rate for next 16 hours
Divide figure in (2) by 16 to give fluid infusion rate
Needs 4200 ml over 16 hours:
   4200/16 = 262.5 ml/hour from 11 pm to 3 pm next day

Maintenance fluid required for a child

A 24 kg child with a resuscitation burn will need the following maintenance fluid:
4 ml/kg/hour for first 10 kg of weight = 40 ml/hour *plus*
2 ml/kg/hour for next 10 kg of weight = 20 ml/hour *plus*
1 ml/kg/hour for next 4 kg of weight = 1×4 kg = 4 ml/hour
Total = 64 ml/hour

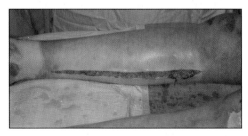

Escharotomy in a leg with a circumferential deep dermal burn

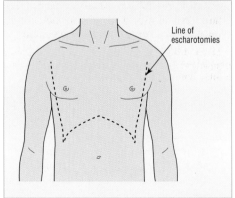

Diagram of escharotomies for the chest

Classification of burn depths

Burns are classified into two groups by the amount of skin loss. Partial thickness burns do not extend through all skin layers, whereas full thickness burns extend through all skin layers into the subcutaneous tissues. Partial thickness burns can be further divided into superficial, superficial dermal, and deep dermal:
- Superficial—The burn affects the epidermis but not the dermis (such as sunburn). It is often called an epidermal burn
- Superficial dermal—The burn extends through the epidermis into the upper layers of the dermis and is associated with blistering
- Deep dermal—The burn extends through the epidermis into the deeper layers of the dermis but not through the entire dermis.

Estimation of burn depth

Assessing burn depth can be difficult. The patient's history will give clues to the expected depth: a flash burn is likely to be superficial, whereas a burn from a flame that was not rapidly extinguished will probably be deep. On direct examination, there are four elements that should be assessed—bleeding on needle prick, sensation, appearance, and blanching to pressure.

Bleeding—Test bleeding with a 21 gauge needle. Brisk bleeding on superficial pricking indicates the burn is superficial or superficial dermal. Delayed bleeding on a deeper prick suggests a deep dermal burn, while no bleeding suggests a full thickness burn.

Sensation—Test sensation with a needle also. Pain equates with a superficial or superficial dermal burn, non-painful sensation equates with deep dermal injury, while full thickness injuries are insensate. However, this test is often inaccurate as oedema also blunts sensation.

Appearance and blanching—Assessing burn depth by appearance is often difficult as burns may be covered with soot or dirt. Blisters should be de-roofed to assess the base. Capillary refill should be assessed by pressing with a sterile cotton bud (such as a bacteriology swab).
- A red, moist wound that obviously blanches and then rapidly refills is superficial
- A pale, dry but blanching wound that regains its colour slowly is superficial dermal
- Deep dermal injuries have a mottled cherry red colour that does not blanch (fixed capillary staining). The blood is fixed within damaged capillaries in the deep dermal plexus
- A dry, leathery or waxy, hard wound that does not blanch is full thickness. With extensive burns, full thickness burns can often be mistaken for unburnt skin in appearance.

Most burns are a mixture of different depths. Assessment of depth is important for planning treatment, as more superficial burns tend to heal spontaneously whereas deeper burns need surgical intervention, but is not necessary for calculating resuscitation formulas. Therefore, in acute situations lengthy depth assessment is inappropriate. A burn is a dynamic wound, and its depth will change depending on the effectiveness of resuscitation. Initial estimates need to be reviewed later.

Competing interests: RP has been reimbursed by Johnson & Johnson, manufacturer of Integra, and Smith & Nephew, manufacturer of Acticoat and TransCyte, for attending symposiums on burn care.

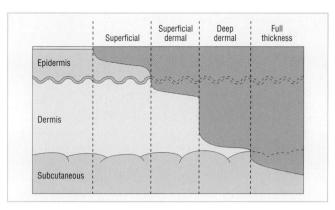

Diagram of the different burn depths

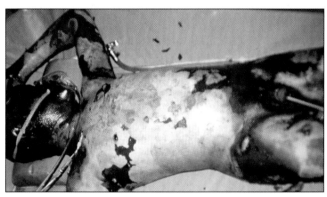

Full thickness burn in a black patient. In a white patient with extensive burns, such full thickness burns can easily be mistaken for unburnt skin

Assessment of burn depth

	Burn type			
	Superficial	Superficial dermal	Deep dermal	Full thickness
Bleeding on pin prick	Brisk	Brisk	Delayed	None
Sensation	Painful	Painful	Dull	None
Appearance	Red, glistening	Dry, whiter	Cherry red	Dry, white, leathery
Blanching to pressure	Yes, brisk return	Yes, slow return	No	No

Key points

- Accurate assessment of burn area is crucial to calculate resuscitation formula
- Resuscitation formulas are only guidelines—monitor the patient
- Discuss resuscitation with a burns unit
- Be aware of the need for escharotomies
- Burn depth is difficult to estimate and changes with resuscitation

Further information

- Clarke J. Burns. *Br Med Bull* 1999;55:885-94
- Herndon D. *Total burn care*. 2nd ed. London: WB Saunders, 2002
- Kao CC, Garner WL. Acute burns. *Plast Reconstr Surg* 2000;105: 2482-93
- Yowler CJ, Fratianne RB. The current status of burn resuscitation. *Clin Plast Surg* 2000;1:1-9
- Collis N, Smith G, Fenton OM. Accuracy of burn size estimation and subsequent fluid resuscitation prior to arrival at the Yorkshire Regional Burns Unit. A three year retrospective study. *Burns* 1999; 25: 345-51
- Burnsurgery.org. www.burnsurgery.org

6   Management of burn injuries of various depths

Remo Papini

Accurate assessment of burn depth on admission is important in making decisions about dressings and surgery. However, the burn wound is a dynamic living environment that will alter depending on both intrinsic factors (such as release of inflammatory mediators, bacterial proliferation) and extrinsic factors (such as dehydration, systemic hypotension, cooling). It is therefore important to review the wound at regular intervals until healing.

Optimum treatment of the wound reduces morbidity and, in larger injuries, mortality. It also shortens the time for healing and return to normal function and reduces the need for secondary reconstruction.

When epithelialisation is delayed beyond three weeks, the incidence of hypertrophic scarring rises. Hypertrophic scars occur in 60% of burnt children aged under 5 years. Early grafting of those burns that have not healed at three weeks has been shown to improve the result, but because of delays in the referral process, all injuries, which show no sign of healing by 10 days, should be referred for assessment.

Treatment

Epidermal burns
By definition these affect only the epidermis and are typified by sunburn. Blistering may occur but is not common. Supportive therapy is usually all that is required, with regular analgesia and intravenous fluids for extensive injuries. Healing occurs rapidly, within a week, by regeneration from undamaged keratinocytes within skin adnexae.

Superficial partial thickness burns
These affect the upper dermis and the epidermis. Blistering is common. The exposed superficial nerves make these injuries painful.

Healing is expected within two weeks by regeneration of epidermis from keratinocytes within sweat glands and hair follicles. The rate of regeneration depends on the density of these skin adnexae: thin hairless skin (inner arm, eyelids, etc) heals more slowly than thick or hairy skin (back, scalp, and face). Progression to a deeper burn is unlikely but can occur if the wound dries out or becomes infected or the patient becomes systemically unwell or hypotensive.

Treatment is aimed at preventing wound progression by the use of antimicrobial creams and occlusive dressings, since epithelialisation progresses faster in a moist environment. Hypafix applied directly to superficial wounds can be useful to preserve mobility and allow washing of the affected part with the dressing intact. It must be soaked in oil (such as olive oil) for an hour before removal, and should be changed at least weekly until the burn has healed.

Alternatively, tulle gras dressing or Mepitel (a silicone dressing) can be applied with or without silver sulfadiazine cream, or Acticoat and gauze, and changed on alternate days. Some burns units treat difficult wounds such as facial burns by leaving them exposed and applying antimicrobial ointment.

If a burn has not healed by two weeks, the depth has probably been assessed incorrectly and referral should be made to a burns unit.

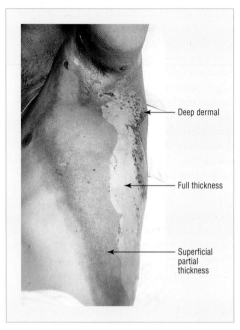

Flame injury showing all burn depths

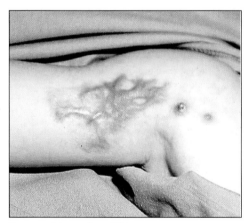

Hypertrophic scar in a child

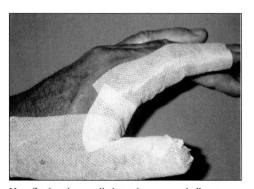

Hypafix dressing applied to a burn wound allows movement and washing

16

Deep partial thickness

These injuries are the most difficult to assess and treat. They may initially seem superficial, with blanching on pressure, but have fixed capillary staining on re-examination after 48 hours. The density of skin adnexae (and hence islands of regeneration) is lower at this depth, and healing is slower and associated with contraction. Therefore, if these injuries are extensive or in functional or cosmetically sensitive areas, they are better excised to a viable depth and then skin grafted to reduce morbidity and to accelerate return to normal function.

Some deep partial thickness injuries will heal if the wound environment is optimised to encourage endogenous healing. This includes keeping it warm, moist, and free of infection. Some of the newer tissue engineered dressings are designed to encourage this by supplying exogenous cytokines. An example is TransCyte, which contains allogeneic non-viable fibroblasts that have produced wound healing factors during manufacture. However, these dressings are highly expensive and need to be applied by trained staff in theatre.

Full thickness injuries

All regenerative elements have been destroyed in these injuries, and healing only occurs from the edges and is associated with considerable contraction. All such injuries should therefore be excised and grafted unless they are < 1 cm in diameter in an area where function would not be compromised.

Timing of surgery

Ideally, all wounds should have epithelial cover within three weeks to minimise scarring, but in practice the decision whether to refer a patient must be made by day 10 to achieve this.

The burn eschar is shaved tangentially or excised to deep fascia. From the surgical viewpoint, the best time to graft burns is within five days of injury to minimise blood loss, and injuries that are obviously deep at presentation must be referred early.

With major burns, treatment is skewed towards preservation of life or limb, and large areas of deep burn must be excised before the burnt tissue triggers multiple organ failure or becomes infected. In such cases more superficial burns may be treated with dressings until healing occurs late or fresh skin donor sites become available.

The ideal covering is split skin autograft from unburnt areas. Thickness is usually tailored to the depth of excision to obtain good cosmesis, although thinner grafts are thought to contract more. Donor sites should ideally be harvested adjacent to the injury to improve colour match, and sheet graft is preferred to improve the cosmetic result.

If donor sites are sparse, however, or the wound bed is likely to bleed profusely (because excision is carried out late, for instance) then the graft is perforated with a mesher to allow expansion. Although this improves graft "take" where the wound bed is bleeding after tangential excision, the mesh pattern is permanent and unsightly. Unmeshed sheet graft is used on hands and faces, and over any future site for intravenous central lines and tracheostomies to obtain rapid cover. Where unburnt split skin donor sites are in very short supply, there are two possible solutions:
● Rotation of donor sites is practised, and unexcised burn covered with antimicrobial creams
● The excised wound is resurfaced with a temporary covering until donor sites have regenerated and can be re-harvested.

Examples of a temporary covering are cadaveric allograft from an unrelated donor, xenograft (such as pigskin), synthetic products, and cultured epithelial autograft. Development of synthetic products (such as Integra dermal regeneration

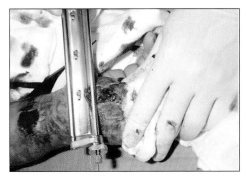
Shave excision to healthy tissue

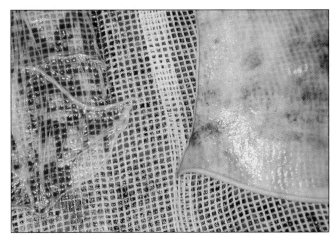
Thick and thin split skin grafts

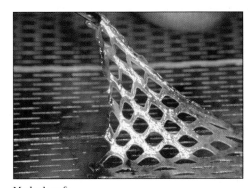
Meshed graft

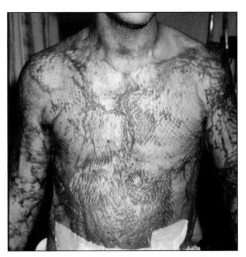
Persistent mesh pattern in patient whose extensive burns were covered with meshed skin grafts

17

template) has allowed us to excise extremely large burns and still achieve physiological closure, with potentially lower mortality in these injuries. Cultured epithelial autografts also permits us to extend the available donor sites. The cultured cells can be applied as sheets (available after three weeks) or in suspension (available within one week). A few burns units use these cells for superficial skin loss or in combination with mesh graft to improve the cosmetic result.

Major burns

These include injuries covering more than 20% of the total body surface area, and represent a real challenge to burn surgeons. Survival depends on accurate assessment and prompt resuscitation initially, as well as on patients' premorbid conditions and associated injuries such as smoke inhalation.

Subsequently, constant attention to wound cleanliness and to nutritional, respiratory, cardiovascular, and renal support is necessary. Relentless but carefully timed removal of burnt tissue and replacement with definitive wound cover is the key to survival and return to function. Such injuries are best managed in large centres where the necessary expertise is concentrated. Early excision and grafting have been shown to reduce pain, shorten hospital stay, and accelerate return to normal function in moderate injuries. It is more difficult to show that this approach improves survival in massive injuries because these are uncommon and many factors other than surgery play a part.

Most major centres treating burns believe early aggressive excision is the treatment of choice, and advances in intensive care and the development of skin substitutes have facilitated this.

Summary

- Full thickness injuries have no regenerative elements left. Unless they are very small they will take weeks to heal and undergo severe contraction. They should be referred for surgery as early as possible.
- Deep dermal injuries are unlikely to heal within three weeks. The incidence of unsightly hypertrophic scarring rises from 33% to 78% if healing is delayed from three to six weeks. Therefore these injuries should also be excised and grafted within the first 5-10 days.
- Superficial wounds should heal by regeneration within two weeks. They should be cleaned, dressed, and reviewed on alternate days to optimise the wound healing environment. Any burn not healed within two weeks should be referred for assessment.
- Clean wounds can be dressed with a non-adherent primary dressing such as tulle gras or Mepitel and an absorbent secondary dressing such as gauze or Gamgee Tissue. Antimicrobial agents are added where infection is likely (perineum, feet) or heavy colonisation is evident on the dressings or invasive infection is suspected.

Competing interests: RP has been reimbursed by Johnson & Johnson, manufacturer of Integra, and Smith & Nephew, manufacturer of Acticoat and TransCyte, for attending symposia on burn care.

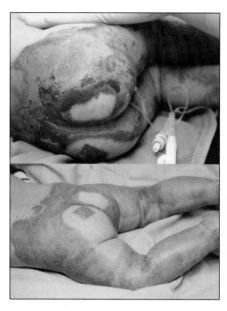

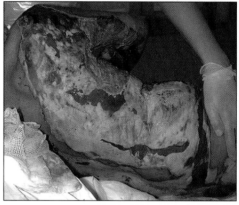

Top: Deep dermal injury from bath scald. Bottom: Six weeks after tangential excision and grafting with 3:1 mesh and cultured epithelial autograft in suspension. Note biopsy site for cell culture on buttock

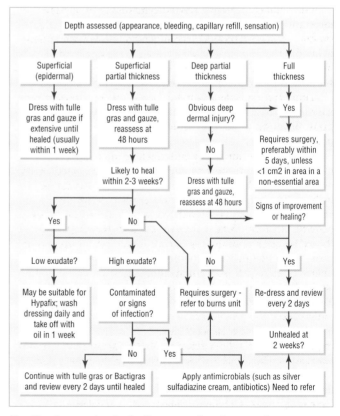

Major burn in elderly patient

Algorithm for assessing depth of burn wounds and suggested treatment

7 Intensive care management and control of infection

Mark Ansermino, Carolyn Hemsley

Intensive care management

The goal in management of an acute burn is to limit the extent of the systemic insult. Intensive care management should not be seen as rescue for failed initial treatment but as a preventive measure in patients at high risk of organ failure. Intensive care units have the resources for improved monitoring and expertise in managing acute physiological changes. Intensive care management should not, however, become an obstacle to early aggressive surgical excision of the burn wound, which is associated with improved outcome.

Airway burns

The term "inhalational injury" has been used to describe the aspiration of toxic products of combustion, but also more generally any pulmonary insult associated with a burn injury. Patients with cutaneous burns are two to three times more likely to die if they also have lower airway burns. Death may be a direct result of lung injury but is usually due to the systemic consequences of such injury. It may be impossible to distinguish lung injury caused at the time of the burn directly to the lungs by a burn from injury due to the systemic consequences of the burn.

Diagnosis of lower airway burns is largely based on the patient's history and clinical examination. Clinicians should have a high index of suspicion of airway burns in patients with one or more of the warning signs. Special investigations will support clinical suspicion. However, severity of injury or prediction of outcome is not aided by additional tests.

The pathophysiology of airway burns is highly variable, depending on the environment of the burn and the incomplete products of combustion. The clinical manifestations are often delayed for the first few hours but are usually apparent by 24 hours. Airway debris—including secretions, mucosal slough, and smoke residue—can seriously compromise pulmonary function.

There is no specific treatment for airway burns other than ensuring adequate oxygenation and minimising iatrogenic lung insult. Prophylactic corticosteroids or antibiotics have no role in treatment.

Control of the airway, by endotracheal intubation, is essential before transporting any patient with suspected airway burn. Rapid fluid administration, with inevitable formation of oedema, may lead to life threatening airway compromise if control of the airway is delayed. Endotracheal intubation before oedema formation is far safer and simpler. Oxygen (100%) should be given until the risk of carbon monoxide toxicity has been excluded, since high concentrations of oxygen will clear carbon monoxide from the body more rapidly than atmospheric concentrations. Importantly, carbon monoxide toxicity may result in a falsely elevated pulse oximetry saturation.

Airway burns are associated with a substantially increased requirement for fluid resuscitation. Reducing the fluid volume administered, to avoid fluid accumulation in the lung, results in a worse outcome. Invasive monitoring may be required to guide fluid administration, especially with failure to respond to increasing volumes of fluid. Adequate oxygen delivery to all the tissues of the body is essential to prevent multi-organ failure.

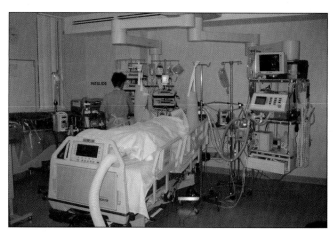

Patient with burns in intensive care unit. Note the bilateral slings raising the burnt hands, air fluidised mattress, warm air heater, haemofiltration, and ventilator

Warning signs of airway burns

Suspect airway burn if:
- Burns occurred in an enclosed space
- Stridor, hoarseness, or cough
- Burns to face, lips, mouth, pharynx, or nasal mucosa
- Soot in sputum, nose, or mouth
- Dyspnoea, decreased level of consciousness, or confusion
- Hypoxaemia (low pulse oximetry saturation or arterial oxygen tension) or increased carbon monoxide levels ($>2\%$)

Onset of symptoms may be delayed

Mechanisms of pulmonary insult after lower airway burns

- Mucosal inflammation
- Mucosal burn
- Bronchorrhoea
- Bronchospasm
- Ciliary paralysis
- Reduced surfactant
- Obstruction by debris
- Systemic inflammatory response

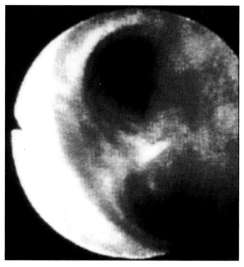

Bronchoscopy image showing mucosal inflammation

Aggressive airway toilet is essential. Diluted heparin and acetyl cystine nebulisation may be helpful. Early surgical debridement, enteral feeding, mobilisation of the patient, and early extubation are desirable. Antibiotics should be reserved for established infections and guided by regular microbiological surveillance.

Several ventilatory strategies have been proposed to improve outcome following airway burns. Adequate systemic oxygenation and minimising further alveolar injury is the primary clinical objective. Prolonging survival will permit spontaneous lung recovery.

Intensive monitoring—The intensive care environment facilitates rapid, graded response to physiological disturbance. Frequent reassessment, based on a range of clinical and monitored parameters, should guide treatment. Fluid administration should not be guided by calculated fluid requirements alone. Failure to respond to treatment should trigger an escalation in the invasiveness of the monitoring.

Heart failure

Myocardial dysfunction is a potential consequence of major burn injury. It has been attributed to a circulating myocardial depressant factor, primarily causing myocardial diastolic dysfunction. It may also be caused by myocardial oedema.

Administration of an inotropic agent is preferable to overloading a failing myocardium with large volumes of fluid. However, the inotropic drug can produce vasoconstriction in the burn wound, reducing the viability of critically injured tissue. Inotropic drugs should not be used until adequate fluid resuscitation has been ensured (usually by invasive monitoring). Inotropic drugs that do not produce vasoconstriction (such as dopexamine or dobutamine) will preserve wound viability, providing they do not produce unacceptable hypotension.

Kidney failure

Early renal failure after burn injury is usually due to delayed or inadequate fluid resuscitation, but it may also result from substantial muscle break down or haemolysis. Delayed renal failure is usually the consequence of sepsis and is often associated with other organ failure.

A reduced urine output, despite adequate fluid administration, is usually the first sign of acute renal failure. This will be followed by a rise in serum creatinine and urea concentrations. Early renal support (haemodialysis or haemodiafiltration) will control serum electrolytes and accommodate the large volumes of nutritional supplementation required in a major burn.

Cerebral failure

Hypoxic cerebral insults and closed head injuries are not uncommonly associated with burn injuries. Fluid administration for the burn injury will increase cerebral oedema and intracranial pressure. Monitoring intracranial pressure may help in minimising the adverse effects of trying to achieve two contradictory treatment goals.

Nutrition

Burn injury is associated with a considerable hypermetabolic response, mediated by the systemic response to the burn and related to the extent of the burn injury. The hypermetabolism may result in a resting energy expenditure increase in excesses of 100% of basal metabolic rate. Even small burns can be associated with hyperpyrexia directly due to hypermetabolism.

Only limited success has been achieved in reducing the hypermetabolic state, which may persist for many months. Close attention to nutritional needs is critical to prevent protein

---

Airway burns—key clinical points

- Restricting fluids increases mortality
- If in doubt, intubate
- Give 100% oxygen until carbon monoxide toxicity excluded
- Ventilatory strategies to avoid lung injury (low volume or pressure)
- Aggressive airway toilet
- Early surgical debridement of wounds
- Early enteral feeding

Possible ventilatory strategies for patients with airway burns

- Low volume ventilation
- Permissive hypercapnia
- High frequency percussive ventilation
- Nitric oxide
- Surfactant replacement
- Partial liquid ventilation (experimental)
- Extracorporeal membrane oxygenation (limited application)

End points to guide fluid administration

- Vital signs (blood pressure, heart rate, capillary refill)
- Urine output
- Peripheral perfusion (temperature gradient)
- Gastric mucosal pH
- Serum lactate or base deficit
- Central venous pressure or pulmonary capillary wedge pressure
- Cardiac output—oxygen delivery and consumption

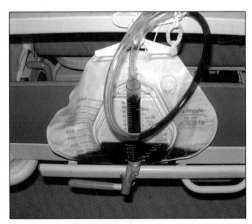

Myoglobinuria in patient after receiving high tension electrical burns

---

Management of the hypermetabolic response

- Reduce heat loss—environmental conditioning
- Excision and closure of burn wound
- Early enteral feeding
- Recognition and treatment of infection

breakdown, decreased wound healing, immune suppression, and an increase in infective complications.

Energy requirements are proportional to the size of the burn and should be met by enteral nutrition, and this should be established as soon as possible after the burn injury. Total parenteral nutrition is associated with immunosuppression, an increase in infective complications, and reduced survival. Glutamine, arginine, and omega 3 fatty acid supplementation may improve immunity and gut function.

Infection in burns patients

After the initial resuscitation, up to 75% of mortality in burns patients is related to infection. Preventing infection, recognising it when it occurs, and treating it successfully present considerable challenges. Infective pulmonary complications are now the commonest types of infection seen in burns patients, but infection is common in many other sites. Several factors contribute to the high frequency and severity of infection at multiple sites in burns patients:
- Destruction of the skin or mucosal surface barrier allows microbial access
- Presence of necrotic tissue and serosanguinous exudate provides a medium to support growth of microorganisms
- Invasive monitoring provides portals for bacterial entry
- Impaired immune function allows microbial proliferation.

Deciding whether infection is present can be difficult. Burns patients have an inflammatory state from the injury itself that can mimic infection. Extensive microbial colonisation of wounds makes interpretation of surface cultures difficult. Patients may have open wounds and repeated episodes of infection over weeks. Excessive use of antibiotics will encourage the appearance of resistant colonising organisms. A sensible approach is to limit antibiotic use to short courses of drugs with as narrow a spectrum of activity as is feasible.

Pathogenesis

The burn injury destroys surface microbes except for Gram positive organisms located in the depths of the sweat glands or hair follicles. Without prophylactic use of topical antimicrobial agents, the wound becomes colonised with large numbers of Gram positive organisms within 48 hours. Gram negative bacteria appear from three to 21 days after the injury. Invasive fungal infection is seen later.

The microbiology reflects the hospital environment and varies from centre to centre. In general there has been a change in the main infective organisms over time from β haemolytic

---

Tube feeding in burns patients
- In all patients with burns covering more than 20% of total body surface area
- Established during initial resuscitation
- Early enteral feeding improves success in establishing feeding
- Nasojejunal feeding will bypass gastric stasis

Risk factors for pneumonia
- Inhalational injury:
  a) Destruction of respiratory epithelial barrier
  b) Loss of ciliary function and impaired secretion clearance
  c) Bronchospasm
  d) Mucus and cellular plugging
- Intubation
- Circumferential, full thickness chest wall burns Decreased chest wall compliance
- Immobility
- Uncontrolled wound sepsis Can lead to secondary pneumonia from haematogenous spread of organisms from wound

---

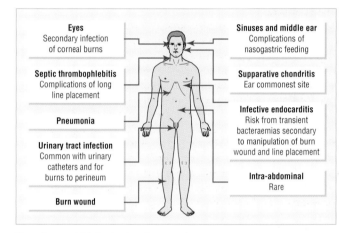

Sites of potential infection in a burns patient

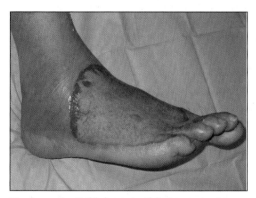

Streptococcal cellulitis in a superficial burn wound

Causative agents of wound infection

Bacteria
β haemolytic streptococci—Such as *Streptococcus pyogenes*. Cause acute cellulitis, and occasionally associated with toxic shock syndrome
Staphylococci—Such as methicillin resistant *Staphylococcus aureus* (MRSA). Cause abscesses and subeschar pus
Gram negative bacteria—Such as *Pseudomonas aeruginosa, Acinetobacter baumanii, Proteus* species. Mini epidemics seen in specialised centres secondary to antibiotic pressure

Fungi
Candida—Most common fungal isolate, act as surface colonisers but have low potential for invasion
Filamentous fungi—Such as *Aspergillus, Fusarium,* and phycomycetes. Can be aggressive invaders of subcutaneous tissues. Treatment must include debridement of infected tissue

Viruses
Herpes simplex—Characterised by vesicular lesions

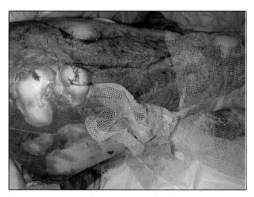

Pseudomonal colonisation of a grafted burn wound on a thigh (note vivid green colouration of dressing)

streptococci to resistant Gram negative organisms including pseudomonas, resistant Gram positive organisms, and fungi.

Preventing invasive wound infection

One aim of initial wound management is to prevent invasive infection. To this end, aggressive surgery and the use of topical antimicrobial agents are effective. Topical antimicrobial treatment slows wound colonisation and is of use early, before definitive surgery. A wide selection of agents are available: silver sulfadiazine is the most frequently used. Early closure of the burn wound by surgical techniques then lessens the surface area available for further microbial colonisation and subsequent infection.

Prophylactic use of systemic antibiotics is controversial. Most agree that prophylactic penicillin against group A streptococcal sepsis is not indicated, and broad spectrum antibiotics to cover wound manipulation are not required in patients with burns covering less than 40% of total body surface area.

Diagnosing invasive wound infection

Surface swabs and cultures cannot distinguish wound infection from colonisation. Wound biopsy, followed by histological examination and quantitative culture, is the definitive method. However, it is time consuming and expensive, making it impractical as a routine diagnostic technique. Diagnosis of infection therefore relies heavily on clinical parameters, with the aid of blood, surface, or tissue cultures to identify likely pathogens.

Treatment

When invasive infection of a burn wound is suspected, empirical systemic antimicrobial treatment must be started. Topical treatment alone is not sufficient, as it does not effectively penetrate the eschar and damaged tissue. The choice of antibiotic depends on the predominant flora on the unit. This can be adjusted later depending on culture and sensitivity results of relevant specimens. Necrotic and heavily infected material must be removed by surgical excision.

Infection control

Infection control measures help to minimise cross infection between patients and acquisition of nosocomial pathogens (such as MRSA or multiresistant Gram negative bacteria). Strict isolation of every patient is impractical, but universal precautions are an absolute necessity.

Advantages and adverse effects of topical antimicrobials

Silver sulfadiazine
- Water soluble cream
- *Advantages*—Broad spectrum, low toxicity, painless
- *Adverse effects*—Transient leucopenia, methaemoglobinaemia (rare)

Cerium nitrate-silver sulfadiazine
- Water soluble cream
- *Advantages*—Broad spectrum, may reduce or reverse immunosuppression after injury
- *Adverse effects*—As for silver sulfadiazine alone

Silver nitrate
- Solution soaked dressing
- *Advantages*—Broad spectrum, painless
- *Adverse effects*—Skin and dressing discolouration, electrolyte disturbance, methaemoglobinaemia (rare)

Mafenide
- Water soluble cream
- *Advantages*—Broad spectrum, penetrates burn eschar
- *Adverse effects*—Potent carbonic anhydrase inhibitor—osmotic diuresis and electrolyte imbalance, painful application

---

Signs of wound infection
- Change in wound appearance:
  a) Discolouration of surrounding skin
  b) Offensive exudate
- Delayed healing
- Graft failure
- Conversion of partial thickness wound to full thickness

Key points
- Fluid resuscitation must be based on frequent reassessment. Formulas are only a guide
- Pulse oximetry readings may be normal in carbon monoxide toxicity
- Unnecessary intubation is preferable to systemic hypoxia
- Early enteral nutrition in major burns may improve survival
- Burn patients are at high risk of infection, and there are many sites for infective complications
- Antibiotics should be used wisely to limit emergence of multiresistant organisms: close liaison with a clinical microbiologist is crucial

---

Further reading
- Still JM Jr, Law EJ. Primary excision of the burn wound. *Clin Plast Surg* 2000;27:23-8
- Desai MH, Mlcak R, Richardson J, Nichols R, Herndon DN. Reduction in mortality in pediatric patients with inhalation injury with aerosolized heparin/N-acetylcystine [correction of acetylcystine] therapy. *J Burn Care Rehabil* 1998;19:210-2
- Pruitt BA, Mc Manus AT, Kim SH, Goodwin MD. Burn wound infections. *World J Surg* 1998;22:135-45
- Monafo WM, West MA. Current treatment recommendations for topical therapy. *Drugs* 1990;40:364-73
- Warren S, Burke JF. Infection of burn wounds: evaluation and management. *Curr Clin Top Infect Dis* 1991;11:206-17

8   Burns reconstruction

Juan P Barret

The basic concerns in burns reconstruction are for function, comfort, and appearance. Normal and hypertrophic scarring, scar contracture, loss of parts of the body, and change in colour and texture of injured skin are processes common to all seriously burnt patients and yet unique to each.

A realistic approach is necessary to harmonise patients' expectations (which are very high) with the probable outcomes of reconstructive surgery. Burn reconstruction starts when a patient is admitted with acute burns and lasts until the patient's expectations have been reached or there is nothing else to offer. However, even when this time has come, the patient-surgeon relationship may still continue and can last a lifetime.

Any surgeon undertaking burn reconstruction must have good understanding of wound healing and scar maturation to plan the time of reconstruction, and sound knowledge of all surgical techniques and all the aftercare required (usually in conjunction with a burn team). A strong patient-surgeon relationship is necessary in order to negotiate a master plan and agree on priorities.

Time of reconstruction

Definitive correction of burn scarring should generally be delayed for a year or more after scar healing. Unsightly scars mature over time, and, with the help of pressure and splints, many of them do not require surgery once the acute phase of scar maturation is over. Patience is often the best tool of a reconstructive surgeon. However, certain problems must be dealt with before scar maturation is complete. In burn reconstruction there are urgent procedures, others that are essential, and many that are desirable. It is for the last group that a good patient-surgeon relationship is necessary for negotiation on which procedures take priority.

Urgent procedures—Waiting for scar maturation is inappropriate when it is certain that an operation is needed to correct a deformity or if vital structures are exposed or can be severely damaged. Urgent procedures should be restricted to those needed to correct function for injuries that are not suitable for other treatments. Examples include an eyelid release to protect an exposed cornea, correction of distracted or entrapped neurovascular bundles, severe fourth degree contractures, and severe microstomia.

Essential procedures—Although they are not urgent since no important structure or the patient's overall health is challenged, essential procedures may, if performed early, improve the patient's final appearance and rehabilitation. Such procedures include operations for all burn scar contractures that do not respond to rehabilitation, and hypertrophic scarring and contractures that prevent a patient from eating, bathing, moving, or performing everyday activities.

Desirable reconstructive procedures—Most of the problems that patients may present fall in this category. These are often aesthetic problems and scars contractures that, although not prominent, produce great discomfort. For all desirable procedures, it is good practice to wait until all red and immature scars have disappeared before starting any kind of surgery. An early operation is often unnecessary in these circumstances.

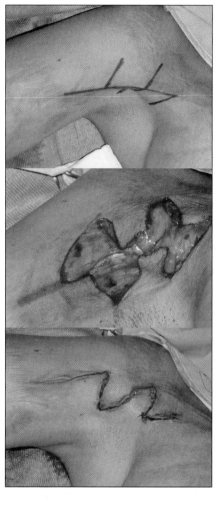

Top: Burn scar contracture on the anterior axillary line. Planned Z-plasties for contracture release are shown.
Middle: The scar has been incised and all flaps raised.
Bottom: Closure of the Z-plasties after rotation of all flaps. Note that the scar contracture has been released and the scar lengthened. This method increases the tissue availability in the reconstructed area and increases the range of motion

---

Techniques for use in acute phase of scar maturation to diminish reconstructive needs

- Use of darts in escharotomies when crossing joints
- Use sheet grafts when possible
- Use aesthetic units to face and hands with medium thickness split skin grafts
- Use of splints, face masks, and silicone inserts as soon as possible
- Place seams following skin tension lines
- Place grafts transversely over joints
- Early pressure therapy
- Early ambulation and exercise

Timing of burn reconstructive surgery

Urgent procedures
- Exposure of vital structures (such as eyelid releases)
- Entrapment or compression of neurovascular bundles
- Fourth degree contractures
- Severe microstomia

Essential procedures
- Reconstruction of function (such as limited range of motion)
- Progressive deformities not correctable by ordinary methods

Desirable procedures
- Reconstruction of passive areas
- Aesthetics

Patient-surgeon relationship

The relationship between a burns patients and a reconstructive burn surgeon is normally long lasting, often continuing for a lifetime. Patients not only require a surgeon's professional expertise, but also time, a good dose of optimism, and compassion.

The initial meeting is one of the most important events. The patient presents a set of problems, and the reconstructive surgeon has to evaluate these and the patient's motivation for surgery and psychological status. We have to remember, though, that the patient will also evaluate the surgeon's attitude and conduct.

Although deformities or chief complaints will often be apparent and ready for surgery, it is preferable to have further visits before surgery, to allow new queries to be addressed and unhurried preparation for surgery. Photographic workup is extremely important to assist in definitive preoperative planning and for documentation.

Patients need frequent reassurance. A reconstructive surgeon needs to know a patient's fears and feelings as the reconstructive plan goes on. A burn reconstruction project commonly requires more than 10 operations and many clinic visits over a long period before a final assessment is made. In the case of a small child, this may take more than 18 years. Patients' feelings and impressions must be addressed continuously, and any trouble, minor disappointment, or depression detected early and treated as needed.

Burn reconstructive visit

One of the most important events during burn reconstruction is the burn reconstructive visit. At that time, a complete and accurate overview of the problems and possible solutions is performed in the following step wise manner:

• Obtain as complete a record of the acute hospitalisation as possible
• Take a thorough history and make a full physical examination
• Make a complete record of all encountered problems. Note quality and colour of the skin in the affected areas—abnormal scars, hyperpigmentation or hypopigmentation, contractures, atrophy, and open wounds
• Consider function. Explore all affected joints and note ranges of motion. Outline any scar contracture extending beyond joints
• Consider skeletal deformities. Scar contractures may distract joints and the body maintain an abnormal position to overcome the deformity. This is particularly true in children; the effect of traction on a growing joint and bone can create long term deformities
• Consider needs for physiotherapy, occupational therapy, and pressure garments. If any of these devices will be needed after surgery the patient must be referred to the rehabilitation department for consideration
• Make an inventory of all possible sites for donor tissue.

Once a patient has voiced all his or her chief complaints and a thorough examination of the patient has been done, a master plan is developed. All reconstructive possibilities are discussed with the patient, and the timing and order of such procedures are outlined.

Surgical procedures

Burn reconstructive surgery has advanced in recent decades, though not as dramatically as in other areas of plastic surgery. For many years, burn reconstructive surgery comprised incisional or excisional releases of scars and skin autografting. Nowadays, however, the first approach that should be considered is use of local or regional flaps. These provide new

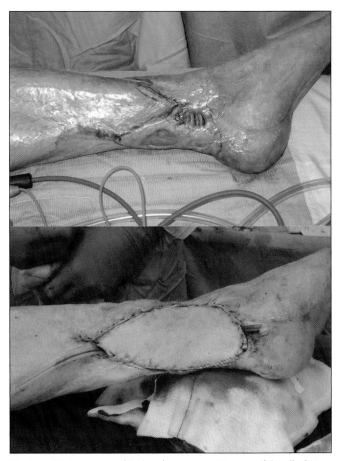

Top: Unstable burn scars with chronic open wounds on medial malleolus. Bottom: The scars were excised and the defect reconstructed with a free vascularised perforator based skin flap. In this case skin from the thigh was transplanted to the ankle with microsurgical vascular anastomosis. These techniques allow the transplantation of any tissue (skin, fascia, fat, functional muscle, and bone) in the same patient

Essentials of burn reconstruction

• Strong patient-surgeon relationship
• Psychological support
• Clarify expectations
• Explain priorities
• Note all available donor sites
• Start with a "winner" (easy and quick operation)
• As many surgeries as possible in preschool years
• Offer multiple, simultaneous procedures
• Reassure and support patient

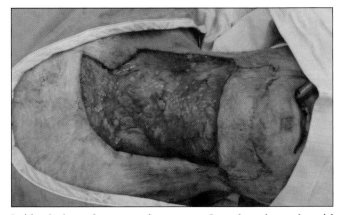

Incisional release of a severe neck contracture. Scar releases leave substantial tissue losses that require extensive skin autografting. Although scar release is still the first choice for some difficult contractures, flap reconstruction and mobilisation of adjacent tissues should be attempted to decrease the size of the defect to be grafted and vascularised tissue to the area, they grow in children, and they give the best functional and cosmetic results. Such flaps can be raised either with normal skin or with burn scar. Even though burnt tissue generally has a high tendency to congestion, ischaemia, and necrosis, it can be used as a reliable flap if extreme care is taken while raising the flap and the injured skin is left attached to the underlying tissues.

When planning surgery for a burnt patient, a surgeon must consider what is the patient's primary complaint, what tissues are left, what parts are missing, and what sort of donor sites are available. This will help to determine the techniques available for burn reconstruction. The patient's chief complaint or complaints need to be carefully evaluated. If immature scars or an increasing deformity is present, and no urgent or essential procedure is required, pressure garments and occupational and physical therapy are indicated. If the deformity is stable and there is a need for reconstruction, an inventory of donor sites and priorities should be made.

Dealing with deficiency of tissue

At this point, the burn injury must be assessed for deficiency in tissue. If there is no deficiency and local tissues can be easily mobilised, excision and direct closure or Z-plasties can be performed.

If, however, there is a deficiency in tissue, the problem of how to reconstruct underlying structures must be addressed. If the deformity affects the skin and subcutaneous tissues, skin autografting, Z-plasties, and all the modifications of them (such as trident flaps) are advised. When reconstruction of underlying structures is necessary, flaps should be considered, including direct cutaneous, musculocutaneous, perforator based, and expanded flaps and microvascular transfer of tissues (free flaps). The precise choice is made on an individual basis.

In addition, composite grafts and bone or cartilage grafts are often necessary in order to perform a complete reconstruction. The use of alloplastic materials in these circumstances is not advisable because of their tendency to extrusion.

Summary

Even though incisional or excisional release and skin autografting (with or without use of dermal templates) are still the main techniques used in burn reconstruction, flaps should be used when possible (remember that Z-plasty and its modifications are transposition flaps). The burn reconstruction plan needs to be tailored to the individual patient and the patient's chief complaint, since certain anatomical areas are better suited to some techniques than others.

Further reading

- Herndon DN, ed. *Total burn care.* 2nd ed. London: WB Saunders, 2002
- Engrav LH, Donelan MB. *Operative techniques in plastic and reconstructive surgery. Face burns: acute care and reconstruction.* London: WB Saunders, 1997
- Achauer BM. *Burn reconstruction.* New York: Thiene, 1991
- Barret JP, Herndon DN. *Color atlas of burn care.* London: WB Saunders, 2001
- Brou JA, Robson MC, McCauley RL. Inventory of potential reconstructive needs in the patient with burns. *J Burn Care Rehabil* 1989;10:555-60

Techniques for burn reconstruction

Without deficiency of tissue
- Excision and primary closure
- Z-plasty

With deficiency of tissue
- Simple reconstruction
- Skin graft
- Dermal templates and skin grafts
  Transposition flaps (Z-plasty and modifications)
- Reconstruction of skin and underlying tissues
  Axial and random flaps
  Myocutaneous flaps
  Tissue expansion
- Free flaps
- Prefabricated flaps

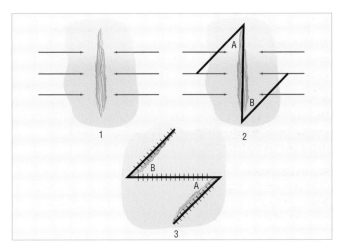

Traditional Z-plasty to release a burn scar contracture. (1) The burn scar, showing the skin tension lines. (2) Z-plasty is performed by rotating two transposition flaps with an angle of 60° with the middle limb of the Z on the scar. (3) Final appearance after insetting of flaps. Note the lengthening of the tissue and the change of scar pattern. Z-plasties can be combined with other flaps (five limb Z-plasty, seven limb Z-plasty, etc)

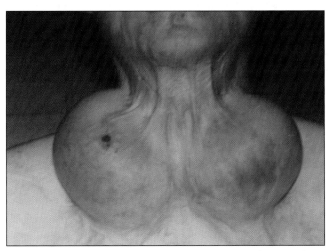

Expansion of normal skin by means of inflatable prostheses implanted in subcutaneous tissue. These are inflated with saline over several weeks until enough extra skin has been created. The expanded skin is then mobilised as full thickness skin grafts, regional advancement flaps, or free flaps. These provide large amounts of normal skin to resurface scarred areas

9 Rehabilitation after burn injury

Dale Edgar, Megan Brereton

Prevention of scarring should be the aim of burn management. For every member of the burn team, rehabilitation must start from the time of injury. Having a substantial burn injury is frightening, particularly as patients will not know what to expect and will be in pain. Consistent and often repetitive education is a vital part of patient care. Oedema management, respiratory management, positioning, and engaging patients in functional activities and movement must start immediately. Patients need to be encouraged to work to their abilities and accept responsibility for their own management. Functional outcome is compromised if patients do not regularly engage in movement.

Pain control

In order to achieve desired outcomes and movement habits, ensuring adequate pain control is important. The aim of analgesic drugs should be to develop a good baseline pain control to allow functional movement and activities of daily living to occur at any time during the day. The use of combined analgesics such as paracetamol, non-steroidal anti-inflammatory drugs, tramadol, and slow release narcotics reduces the need for increasing doses of narcotics for breakthrough pain. Codeine should be avoided if possible because of its negative effects on gut motility. Other pain control methods that may be helpful include transcutaneous electrical nerve stimulation (TENS).

Inhalational injury

Aggressive, prophylactic chest treatment should start on suspicion of an inhalational injury. If there is a history of burn in a closed space or the patient has a reduced level of consciousness then frequent, short treatments should begin on admission. Treatment should be aimed at removing lung secretions (oedema), normalising breathing mechanics, and preventing complications such as pneumonia.
Initial treatment should include:
• Normalisation of breathing mechanics—such as using a positive expiratory pressure device, intermittent positive pressure breathing, sitting out of bed, positioning
• Improving the depth of breathing and collateral alveolar ventilation—such as by ambulation or, when that is not possible, a tilt table, facilitation techniques, inspiratory holds

Movement and function

Movement is a habit that should be encouraged from admission to the burns unit. If a patient can accept the responsibility of self exercise and activities of daily living then the most difficult aspects of rehabilitation are easily achieved. If there is suspected tendon damage from the burn, then protected movement is appropriate and resting splints may be necessary.

Oedema management

Oedema removal should be encouraged from admission. The only body system that can actively remove excess fluid and debris from the interstitium is the lymphatic system. Oedema

Rehabilitation starts on the day of injury

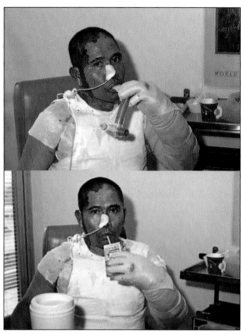

Functional use of a positive expiratory pressure device to improve breathing mechanics (top) and practising activities of daily living to exercise a burnt limb (bottom)

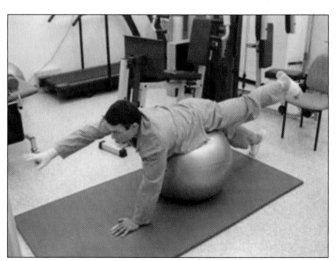

Strengthening exercise for a patient who had sustained a high tension electrical flash burn to the right upper limb and right lateral trunk. Rehabilitation to restore function focuses on upper limb strength and trunk core stability

26

collection in the zone of stasis of a burn may promote the progression of depth of a burn. The principles of reduction of oedema should be adhered to in totality and not just in part:

- Compression—such as Coban, oedema gloves
- Movement—rhythmic, pumping
- Elevation or positioning of limbs for gravity assisted flow of oedema from them
- Maximisation of lymphatic function
- Splinting does not control oedema except to channel fluid to an immobile area.

Immobilisation

Stopping movement, function, and ambulation has its place. It should be enforced only when there is concomitant injury to tendon or bone or when tissues have been repaired (including skin reconstruction). If a body part must be immobilised—to allow skin graft adherence, for example—then the part should be splinted or positioned in an anti-deformity position for the minimum time possible.

Skin reconstruction

Skin reconstruction is tailored to the depth of burn found at the time of surgery. The application and time frames of reconstruction techniques utilised will be dependent on attending surgeon's preference. Other factors influencing choice of management include availability and cost of biotechnological products.

Scar management

Scar management relates to the physical and aesthetic components as well as the emotional and psychosocial implications of scarring.

Hypertrophic scarring results from the build up of excess collagen fibres during wound healing and the reorientation of those fibres in non-uniform patterns.

Keloid scarring differs from hypertrophic scarring in that it extends beyond the boundary of the initial injury. It is more common in people with pigmented skin than in white people.

Scarring is influenced by many factors:

- Extraneous factors—First aid, adequacy of fluid resuscitation, positioning in hospital, surgical intervention, wound and dressing management
- Patient related factors—Degree of compliance with rehabilitation programme, degree of motivation, age, pregnancy, skin pigmentation.

Management techniques

Pressure garments are the primary intervention in scar management. Applying pressure to a burn is thought to reduce scarring by hastening scar maturation and encouraging reorientation of collagen fibres into uniform, parallel patterns as opposed to the whorled pattern seen in untreated scars.

Garments need to be tailored to patients' requirements and are often influenced by the type of surgery completed. Patients should generally be measured for garments at five to seven days after grafting surgery, and these should be fitted as soon as they are available. A pressure garment lasts for about three months; after that time it is helpful to re-measure patients frequently to accommodate the changing dimensions of the scar.

If people have moderate to severe burns around the neck or face, an acrylic face mask must be considered. This provides conforming pressure over the face and neck. Material masks can also be made for patients to wear at night.

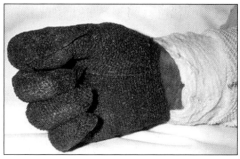
Compression glove (Coban)

Immobilisation times for different types of skin reconstruction

Reconstruction method	Depth of burn	Length of immobilisation
Biological dressings (such as Biobrane, TransCyte)	Any (preferably not full thickness)	<24 hours
Cultured epithelial autograft (suspension)	Superficial to intermediate	24-48 hours
Split skin graft	Intermediate to deep partial thickness	3-5 days
Dermal substitutes (such as Integra, Alloderm)	Deep partial thickness to full thickness	5-7 days
Fasciocutaneous or myocutaneous flaps	Full thickness	7-14 days

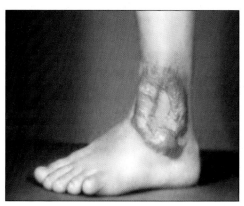
Example of hypertrophic scarring

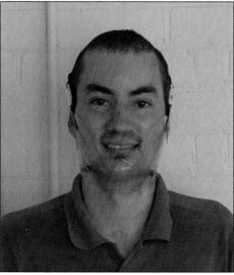
Acrylic face mask providing conforming pressure over burns to the face and neck

For areas of persistent scarring that have not responded well to pressure garments, further scar management techniques must be considered. These include the use of massage, moisturising creams, and contact media.

Team education of scar management

Because of the altered functions of the skin after a burn, patients should be continually encouraged to maintain a good moisturising regimen. Moisturising is important as it prevents the skin from drying out and then splitting and cracking, which may lead to secondary infection and breakdown of the skin.

Education on sun protection is also important for patients. Patients must be made aware that they need to protect themselves from the sun for up to two years and that they will need to keep their skin protected and covered in sun screen (and appropriate clothing) if working or playing outside.

Outpatient follow up

A burns unit team should offer outpatients regular and comprehensive follow up reviews. The type of follow up required obviously depends on the severity of the burn, but in terms of movement and function, patients require regular monitoring and updating of their prescribed exercise regimen and home activity programme.

Therapists who do not regularly treat burns patients require experienced support to achieve the expected outcomes. This should include written, verbal, and visual communications as well as monitoring of management plans.

Conclusion

The rehabilitation of burns patients is a continuum of active therapy. There should be no delineation between an "acute phase" and a "rehabilitation phase"—instead, therapy needs to start from the day of admission (and before if possible). Education is of paramount importance to encourage patients to accept responsibility for their rehabilitation. A consistent approach from all members of the multidisciplinary team facilitates ongoing education and rehabilitation.

Further reading

- Schnebly WA, Ward RS, Warden GD, Saffle JR. A nonsplinting approach to the care of the thermally injured patient. *J Burn Care Rehabil* 1989;10:263-6

Scar management techniques in addition to pressure

- Massage—Helps to soften restrictive bands of scar tissue, makes scar areas more pliable
- Silicone gel sheets (contact media)—Mode of action not known; possibly limits the contraction of scars through hydration, occlusion, and low molecular weight silicone
- Elastomer moulds (contact media)—Used to flatten areas of scarring where it is difficult to encourage silicone to mould effectively (such as toes and web spaces between them)
- Hydrocolloids (contact media)—As for silicone sheets, except that these may be left in situ for up to 7 days. Massage can be given through thin sheets
- Moisturising creams—Combined with massage to compensate for lost secretory functions of skin; protect against complications from skin cracking
- Ultrasound—Low pulsed dose aimed at progressing the inflammatory process more rapidly

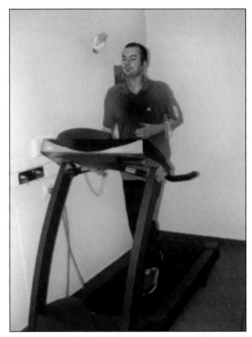

Endurance training by a burns outpatient

10 Psychosocial aspects of burn injuries

Shelley A Wiechman, David R Patterson

With the increased survival of patients with large burns comes a new focus on the psychological challenges and recovery that such patients must face. Most burn centres employ social workers, vocational counsellors, and psychologists as part of the multidisciplinary burn team. Physiological recovery of burn patients is seen as a continual process divided into three stages—resuscitative or critical, acute, and long term rehabilitation. The psychological needs of burn patients differ at each stage.

Resuscitative or critical stage

The psychological characteristics of this stage include stressors of the intensive care environment, uncertainty about outcome, and a struggle for survival. The intensive care environment can be both overstimulating and understimulating with the monotony of lying in a hospital bed for weeks.

Cognitive changes such as extreme drowsiness, confusion, and disorientation are common during this phase. More severe cognitive changes such as delirium and brief psychotic reactions also occur, usually as a result of infections, alcohol withdrawal, metabolic complications, or high doses of drugs. Patients may also be intubated, which greatly limits direct communication.

Treatment

In depth psychological intervention is of minimal value at this phase, since physical survival is the primary goal. Patients should be encouraged to cope with the frighteningly unusual circumstances of the intensive care unit through whatever defences are available to them, even primitive strategies such as denial and repression. Supportive psychological interventions should focus on immediate concerns, such as sleep, pain control, and protecting patients' coping strategies. Non-pharmacological approaches to pain control, such as hypnosis and relaxation, can be effective.

Medical staff can also effectively intervene during this early stage of recovery by working with a patient's family members. Family members may be anxious and distressed while observing the patient undergo treatment, which fosters the same response in the patient. It is important to help family members understand this effect and help them to convey a sense of hope and calmness to the patient.

Acute stage

The acute phase of recovery focuses on restorative care, but patients continue to undergo painful treatments. As patients become more alert during this phase, they face these procedures with less sedation. Also, patients are more aware of the physical and psychological impact of their injuries.

Depression and anxiety—Symptoms of depression and anxiety are common and start to appear in the acute phase of recovery. Acute stress disorder (occurs in the first month) and post-traumatic stress disorder (occurs after one month) are more common after burns than other forms of injury. Patients with these disorders typically have larger burns and more severe pain and express more guilt about the precipitating event. The severity of depression is correlated with a patient's level of resting pain and level of social support.

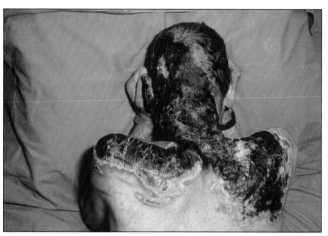

With the increased survival of patients with large burns, there is increased focus on the psychological challenges and recovery that such patients must face

The psychological needs of patients with burn injuries are unique at each stage of physical recovery

---

Psychological characteristics of critical stage of recovery from a burn

Challenges
- Overstimulation
- Understimulation
- Delirium, confusion, and disorientation
- Impaired communication
- Sleep disturbance
- Pain

Treatments
- Protect patient's natural defences and coping strategies
- Drug management for pain control and to help with sleep
- Non-pharmacological techniques for pain management
- Educate and provide support to family members
- Educate and provide support to staff

Prevalence of depression and anxiety in inpatients with burns

Condition	Prevalence
Depression	23-61%
Generalised anxiety	13-47%
Post-traumatic stress disorder	30%

Sleep disturbance—Central to both anxiety and depression is sleep disturbance. The hospital environment can be loud, and patients are awakened periodically during the night for analgesia or for checking vital signs. Patients' mood, agitation, and nightmares can all affect sleep.

Premorbid psychopathology—Compared with the general population, burn patients have a high rate of premorbid psychopathology. Patients with pre-existing psychopathology typically cope with hospitalisation through previously established dysfunctional and disruptive strategies. The most common premorbid psychiatric diagnoses are depression, personality disorders, and substance misuse. Prior psychopathology can have an adverse impact on outcomes, including longer hospitalisations and the development of more serious psychopathologies after injury.

Grief—Patients may now begin the grieving process as they become more aware of the impact of the burn injuries on their lives. Family members, friends, or pets may have died in the incident, and patients may have lost their homes or personal property. In addition to these external losses, patients may also grieve for their former life (such as job, mobility, physical ability, appearance). Mental health professionals and other staff should help patients to grieve in their own way and at their own pace.

Treatment

Brief psychological counselling can help both depression and anxiety, but drugs may also be necessary. When offering counselling, it is often helpful to provide reassurance that symptoms often diminish on their own, particularly if the patient has no premorbid history of depression or anxiety.

Drugs and relaxation techniques may also be necessary to help patients sleep. Informing patients that nightmares are common and typically subside in about a month can help allay concerns. Occasionally patients will benefit from being able to talk through the events of the incident repeatedly, allowing them to confront rather than avoid reminders of the trauma. Staff often make the mistake of trying to treat premorbid psychopathology during patients' hospitalisation. Referrals to community treatment programmes should be made once patients are ready for discharge.

Pain control

Both procedural and background pain can be challenging for patients and staff. Some patients report that procedural pain is easier to cope with because of its transient nature, whereas with background pain there is no clear end in sight. It is important to conduct a thorough pain assessment in order to determine which type of pain is the greatest problem.

A pain treatment plan that provides pharmacological and non-pharmacological approaches should be established. Opioid agonists are the most commonly used analgesics. Long acting opiates are used for background pain, and short acting opiates are used for painful procedures such as wound care. It is crucial that drugs for background pain are provided on a fixed dose schedule to maintain control of the pain. Opioid analgesics may be supplemented with other drugs, including inhaled nitrous oxide and anxiolytics. Lorazepam has recently been found to lessen burn pain, largely by treating acute anxiety.

Non-pharmacological pain control techniques include cognitive-behaviour therapy and hypnosis. These have been shown to be effective in treating procedural pain. One exciting new distraction technique is virtual reality. Since attentional focus is limited and a person cannot attend to more than one stimulus at a time, virtual reality creates a realistic environment for patients to absorb themselves in during painful procedures, thus taking focus away from the discomfort.

Psychological characteristics of acute stage of recovery from a burn

Challenges
- Pain—both background and procedural
- Anxiety—both acute stress disorder and post-traumatic stress disorder
- Depression
- Sleep disturbance
- Premorbid psychopathology becomes more apparent
- Grief

Treatments
- Drug management of anxiety, pain, sleeplessness, and depression
- Brief counselling
- Teach non-drug approaches to pain management (relaxation, imagery, hypnosis, virtual reality)

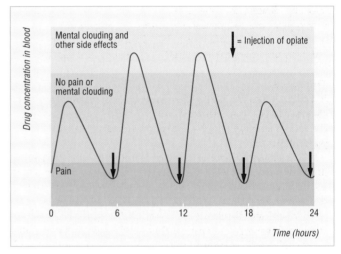

Effects of fixed dose schedule of analgesic drugs for pain control

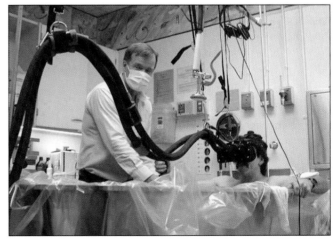

A patient's attention is taken up with "SnowWorld" via a water-friendly virtual reality helmet during wound care in the hydrotub

Long term rehabilitation

The long term stage of recovery typically begins after discharge from hospital, when patients begin to reintegrate into society. For patients with severe burns, this stage may involve continued outpatient physical rehabilitation, possibly with continuation of procedures such as dressing changes and surgery. This is a period when patients slowly regain a sense of competence while simultaneously adjusting to the practical limitations of their injury. The first year after hospitalisation is a psychologically unique period of high distress.

Physical problems—Patients face a variety of daily hassles during this phase, such as compensating for an inability to use hands, limited endurance, and severe itching. Severe burn injuries that result in amputations, neuropathies, heterotopic ossification, and scarring can have an emotional and physical effect on patients.

Psychosocial problems—In addition to the high demands of rehabilitation, patients must deal with social stressors including family strains, return to work, sexual dysfunction, change in body image, and disruption in daily life. Many people continue to have vivid memories of the incident, causing distress. Patients may also develop symptoms of depression. There is evidence that adjustment to burn injuries improves over time independent of the injury size. Social support is an important buffer against the development of psychological difficulty.

Treatment

It can be helpful to make follow up telephone calls to patients after discharge or to continue to see patients in an outpatient clinic to screen for symptoms of distress and to provide psychotherapy.

Adjustment difficulties that persist more than a year after discharge usually involve perceptions of a diminished quality of life and lowered self esteem. Some studies suggest that burn disfigurement in general leads to decreased self esteem in women and social withdrawal in men. "Changing Faces" is a successful programme for enhancing self esteem. This includes a hospital based programme for image enhancement and social skills plus a series of publications for patients dealing with aspects of facial disfigurement.

Many patients face a lengthy period of outpatient recovery before being able to return to work. Some patients go through vocational challenges. In a recent study of patients hospitalised for burn injury 66% returned to work within six months of their injury, and 81% had returned by one year. As expected, patients who sustained larger burns took longer to return to work. About half of the patients required some change in job status.

Ancillary resources such as support groups and peer counselling by burn survivors can also be important services to burn survivors. Major burn centres ideally have a network of burn survivors who are willing to talk with patients in the hospital.

Summary

A burn injury and its subsequent treatment are among the most painful experiences a person can encounter. The emotional needs of patients with burns have long been overshadowed by the emphasis on survival. Patients undergo various stages of adjustment and face emotional challenges that parallel the stage of physical recovery. Adjustment to a burn injury seems to involve a complex interplay between the patient's characteristics before the injury, moderating environmental factors, and the nature of the injury and ensuing medical care.

The picture of a patient with burnt head and shoulders is reproduced with permission of Science Photo Library.

Psychological characteristics during rehabilitation stage of recovery from a burn

Challenges

Physical—Itching, limited endurance, decrease in function

Social—Changing roles, return to work, body image, sexual issues

Psychological—Anxiety, depression

Treatments
- Outpatient counselling
- Social skills training
- Support groups
- Peer counselling
- Vocational counselling

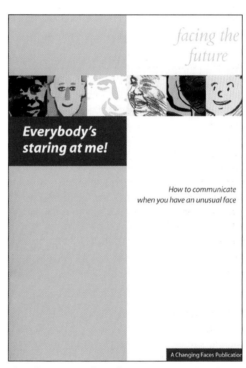

Changing Faces (United Kingdom) and the Phoenix Society (United States) are excellent sources of information and support for burn survivors

---

Further reading
- Patterson DR, Everett JJ, Bombardier CH, Questad KA, Lee VK, Marvin JA. Psychological effects of severe burn injuries. *Psychol Bull* 1993;113:362-78
- Patterson DR, Ford GR. Burn injuries. In: Frank RG, Elliott TT, eds. *Handbook of rehabilitation psychology*. Washington DC: American Psychological Association, 2000:145-62
- Partridge J. *When burns affect the way you look*. London: Changing Faces, 1997

11   Burns in the developing world and burn disasters

Rajeev B Ahuja, Sameek Bhattacharya

Burns in the developing world

Developing countries have a high incidence of burn injuries, creating a formidable public health problem. High population density, illiteracy, and poverty are the main demographic factors associated with a high risk of burn injury. The exact number of burns is difficult to determine: judicious extrapolation suggests that India, with a population of over 1 billion, has 700 000 to 800 000 burn admissions annually. The high incidence makes burns an endemic health hazard. Social, economic, and cultural factors interact to complicate the management, reporting, and prevention of burns.

Epidemiology

The epidemiology of burn injuries is different from that in the developed world. Most burn injuries are sustained by women aged 16-35 years. Women of this age group tend to be engaged in cooking, and most work at floor level in relatively unsafe kitchens and wear loose fitting clothes such as saris, dupatta, etc. Children and elderly people are at relatively less risk because many households still exist as joint families, and the system safeguards these age groups to some extent.

The commonest mode of burn injury is a flame burn. Most such incidents are related to malfunctioning kerosene pressure stoves. These are cheap contraptions without safety features, and burns occur when carbon deposits block the kerosene vapour outlets. Unsupervised and careless handling of firecrackers during the festival of Diwali lead to an increased incidence of injuries during the festival period. Fire is also used in homicide and suicide.

Problems in management

Burn management in developing countries is riddled with difficulties. Lack of government initiative and low literacy rates preclude effective prevention programmes. Many uneducated households are fraught with superstition, taboos, weird religious rituals, and faith in alternative systems of "medicine," which complicates management.

Most burn centres are situated in large cities and are inadequate for the high incidence of injuries. Resuscitation is often delayed as patients have to travel long distances and transport facilities are poor. Many burn centres are also plagued with lack of resources, lack of operating time, and shortage of blood. Often there are no dedicated burn surgeons, and general surgeons without formal training are involved in burn care. Burn nursing is also not a recognised concept. These conditions make excisional surgery impossible for a large percentage of patients. There is generally no coordination between district hospitals and tertiary burn centres.

Strategies for effective burn care in developing countries

The approach to burn management has to be radically different from that in Western countries.

Prevention programmes

Prevention programmes should be directed at behavioural and environmental changes which can be easily adopted into lifestyle. The programmes need to be executed with patience, persistence, and precision, targeting high risk groups.

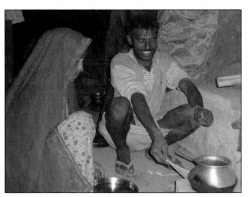

Cooking at floor level in loose fitting clothes such as "dupatta" places women at increased risk of burn injury

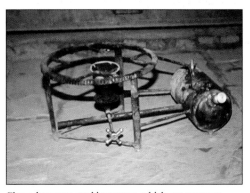

Cheap kerosene cooking stoves, which are prone to malfunction, are a common cause of burns

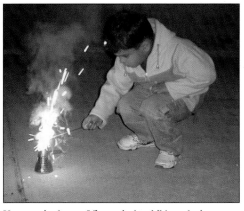

Unsupervised use of fireworks by children during festivals such as Diwali increases the incidence of burns during the festival period

Burn management problems in developing countries

- High incidence of burns
- Lack of prevention programmes
- Inadequate burn care facilities
- Lack of resources
- Lack of trained staff
- Poor infrastructure and coordination
- Social problems

Depending on the population of the country, burns prevention could be a national programme. This can ensure sufficient funds are available and lead to proper coordination of district, regional, and tertiary care centres. It could also provide for compulsory reporting of all burn admissions to a central registry, and these data could be used to evaluate strategies and prevention programmes. There should be adequate provision by law to set manufacturing standards for heating and electrical equipment, fire safety standards for high rise buildings, and procedures for storage and transportation of hazardous materials, explosive chemicals, and firecrackers. A national body of burn professionals should be constituted to educate all healthcare staff involved in burn care.

Providing treatment
To provide optimal burn care to a large population with limited resources, it is imperative to strengthen the existing infrastructure. A few regional burn centres should be developed to provide tertiary management and training to burn care staff. General surgeons working in district hospitals should form the nucleus of the burn care service and decide on referral procedures.

If it is not possible to keep referred patients at burn centres for six to eight weeks of treatment, they can be discharged after two or three weeks of stabilisation. Such patients can then be treated at district hospitals or at home with the help of primary health centres. Thus, primary health centres can act as liaison between burn patients and district hospitals. The incidence of burn wound septicaemia with domiciliary treatment is remarkably low. These patients can be readmitted as necessary for blood transfusions, treating septicaemia, and skin grafting.

Certain well tested and cost effective treatment procedures need to be adopted to conserve resources: these include using Parkland formula for resuscitation, pursuing conservative burn wound management, and using amnion as a biological dressing.

Burn disasters

A disaster is a situation that is unpredictable, massive, and poses an immediate threat to public health. A burn disaster is "an event resulting in mass burn casualties and severe loss of human lives and material from a known thermal agent." Disasters normally exceed the resources of local healthcare facilities.

Disaster management involves coordinating the activities of various health disciplines to prevent disasters, provide an immediate response to a disaster, and help in rehabilitation of victims.

Disaster plan
An organised disaster plan can reduce loss of property, social disruption, and suffering. A disaster plan should be specifically tailored for a particular region and nature of fire disaster. Ultimately, a coordinated system must be developed that includes medical and public safety organisations, law and order agencies, and transport agencies.

The communication lines from the central command should be fast and multilingual. It should be able to advise workers at the disaster site, direct transport agencies, and simultaneously relay the information to surrounding hospitals. All the regional and distant hospitals must be incorporated in a multi-tier system as the number of cases may overwhelm local facilities.

Hospitals play a pivotal role in providing trained staff. All doctors and nurses, irrespective of their specialties and whether they are included in the plan, should be educated about the basics of burn care. With a burn specialist at the core, the

---

Strategies for burn management in developing countries

- Effective prevention programmes
- Burns as national health agenda
- Central registry of burns
- Create a professional burn group
- Adequate safety legislation
- Induct district hospitals and primary health centres
- Encourage patient management at home
- Cost effective treatment procedures
- Develop regional centres of excellence

Cost effective burn treatments to conserve scare resources

Parkland formula for fluid resuscitation
This is cost effective and ensures proper compliance

Conservative burn wound management
This involves using closed dressings, eschar separation, and skin grafting. This takes the pressure off operating facilities and provides comparable results to surgery

Amnion as a biological dressing
This is easily available, is free of cost, and can be comfortably preserved for a week

---

Characteristics of a burn disaster

- Large number of patients with extensive burn injuries
- A high incidence of serious associated injuries
- Site of the disaster is not always accessible
- Immediate care and assistance may not be adequate
- Response time may be prolonged
- Local infrastructure may be affected by fire

Principles of disaster management

- Prevention
- Disaster profiles
- Disease patterns
- Risk assessment
- Post-emergency phase
- Effective multidisciplinary response
- Mobilisation of workforce resources
- Local community or national involvement
- Reconstructive phase

Factors to be considered while developing a disaster plan

- Unpredictability
- Characteristics (explosion, building fire, toxic fumes, etc)
- Type of building (dwelling, hotel, office, etc)
- Type of trauma (burn, associated injury, inhalational injury)
- Time (day, night, during festivities, etc)
- Area (city, non-urban, accessibility, etc)
- Number of people injured
- Degree of preparedness to manage a disaster

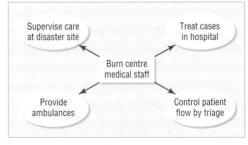

Role of hospital in disaster management

hospital disaster management team also includes a respiratory physician and an anaesthetist. There should be prompt and judicious deployment of staff. Teams of psychologists should manage panic among disaster victims and their relatives both at the disaster site and at hospitals. Accurate triage by clinicians experienced in burns must guide the flow of patients from the site to the inner circle of healthcare facilities (primary and secondary care hospitals) and then to the outer circle (tertiary care hospitals and burn centres).

Transportation needs are guided by the number of victims, their condition, the nature of the fire disaster, and geographical considerations. Possible modes of transport include ambulances, local transport vehicles, military vehicles, helicopters, fixed wing aircraft, and rescue boats.

Managing a disaster

Immediate care is provided by people present at the scene of the disaster, who may be survivors or passers by. These first responders are later guided by trained healthcare workers who arrive at the site. On site management includes first aid, patient triage, and ambulance staging with a basic aim of maximal use of resources.

Triage

Triage is the cornerstone of effective burn disaster management and is done at the disaster site by staff with knowledge of burn treatment. Triage takes into consideration the total number of patients, bed availability, and transportation capacity.

Triage should be prognostic, and patients should be categorised on the basis of age, extent of burns, site of burns and presence of inhalational injury:

- *Group I*—Minor burns (< 10% of total surface area in children, < 20% in adults) to non-critical areas
  Assigned to—Outpatient care, dressing, tetanus prophylaxis
- *Group II*—Minor burns to critical sites (face, hands, genitalia)
  Assigned to—Short hospital stay, special wound care or operation
- *Group III*—Major burns (20-60%)
  Assigned to—Admission to burn unit, intravenous resuscitation
- *Group IV*—Extensive burns (>60%)
  Assigned to—Lower priority for transfer
- *Group V*—Minor burns with inhalational injury or associated injury
  Assigned to—Oxygen, intubation, transfer to intensive care unit.

The patients in groups III and V are evacuated first, followed by group IV. Group II cases are evacuated at the end. Group I cases are either discharged after first aid or asked to make their own way to the nearest primary care centre.

Further treatment

Initial care is in the line of ABC of resuscitation. An adequate airway and respiration must be ensured. All patients except those with minor burns must receive fluid resuscitation based on a simple formula. Wounds should be covered with a sterile sheet until they are dressed. Dressings should be simple, with only antimicrobial pads and Gamgee Tissue. Effort should be made to detect and treat associated injuries.

Secondary triage may also be done at this time. If necessary, seriously injured patients can be sent to centres of higher level while less serious patients who reach the tertiary centres are referred back to primary care centres. The success of such a plan lies in accurate triage at every level, so that all centres are used optimally and best possible treatment is delivered to all according to the severity of injury, with minimum delay.

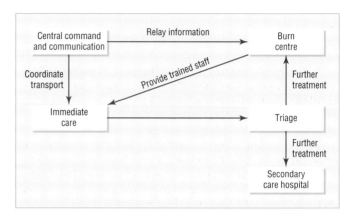

Major arms of a disaster plan

First aid at the site of a burn disaster

- Quantitative assessment of burns
- Qualitative assessment of burns
- Commence intravenous resuscitation
- Catheterisation
- Analgesia
- Hospital transfer

Further reading

Burns in the developing world

- Davies JWL. The problem of burns in India. *Burns* 1990;17(suppl 1):S2-22
- Sawhney CP, Ahuja RB, Goel A. Burns in India: epidemiology and problems in management. *Ind J Burns* 1993;1:1-4
- Ahuja RB. Managing burns in India—focussing on newer strategies. *Ind J Burns* 1995;3:1-7
- Ahuja RB, Bhattacharya S. An analysis of 11 196 burn admissions and evaluation of conservative management techniques. *Burns* 2002;28:555-61

Burn disasters

- Watchel TL, Dimick AR. Burn disaster management. In: Herndon DN, ed. *Total burn care.* Philadelphia: WB Saunders, 1998:19-32
- Hadjiiski O. Behaviour during a mass industrial burn disaster. *Ann Burn Fire Disaster* 1996;9:232-7
- Masellis M, Gunn SWA. Thermal agent disaster and burn disaster: definition, damage, assessment and relief operation. *Ann Burn Fire Disaster* 1991;4:215-9

12　When we leave hospital: a patient's perspective of burn injury

Amy Acton

At the age of 18, I thought I had the best summer job possible, working outside at the local marina, with the prospect of going to college in a few months to become a nurse. In an instant everything changed. While moving a boat on a trailer, a group of us sustained electrical injuries when the mast hit a high tension power line. I found myself fighting for my life in a burns centre and mourning the loss of a friend. The physical healing was gruelling and at times overwhelming for me and my family, and the medical team was a great support for me. However, this article focuses on the problems I faced once I left the hospital, two and a half months later, because that was toughest part of my journey.

My comments are both personal and from the perspective of having been a burn nurse for over 13 years. It is a shared story of healing the emotional scars of burn injuries because I have learnt so much from others. One such person is Barbara Kammerer Quayle, a fellow burn survivor and colleague I met after I became a burn nurse. She taught me how healthcare professionals could make a difference for survivors struggling to regain a place in their family and society. Many of the strategies I discuss are her life's work and are used with her permission. For some burn survivors these strategies are natural responses, but for others they have to be learnt and practised.

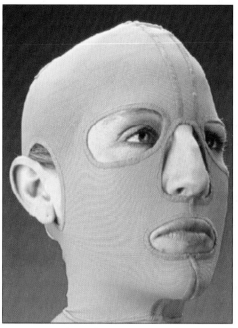

Pressure garments stimulate reactions such as stares and questions

Facing the world

While in the secure cocoon of the burn centre, I received extraordinary social support and acceptance from staff. After my discharge and return to my community, however, I felt surprised, shocked, and sometimes completely overwhelmed as I realised I would face the curious stares of strangers. I had remained focused on my physical healing and had never thought about how my burns would affect my life long term. Addressing this issue with patients and families must become part of the discharge process from burns centres.

Before my burn injury, I passed through shops, restaurants, churches, and social occasions with minimal interest from others. Now, wearing splints and pressure garments, I found all of that had changed. I was not prepared for this and had no idea of how to cope with people's reactions. It was not until almost two years later that I felt comfortable in social settings, as I learnt to love my body again and realised that I could make a big difference to how others responded by my attitude.

Attitudes about appearance

From childhood onward, we develop our attitudes about appearance. We possess a complex set of beliefs about what appearance means in our life. These beliefs are the result of our thoughts and influences by parents, teachers, friends, magazines, films, and television.

When my appearance was altered by my burns it threatened my existing thoughts and beliefs about my appearance and who I was. Over time, I and many other burn survivors do accept the alteration in our appearance, and incorporate the changes into a healthy body image, and go on to live successful lives. This takes time, support, self love, and learning new behavioural skills. For some, it is a lifelong struggle.

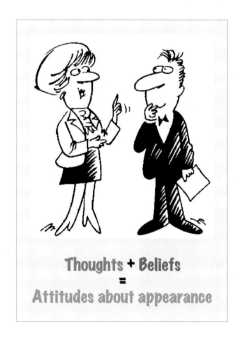

Thoughts + Beliefs = Attitudes about appearance

Staring: a fact of life

Staring is part of human nature. Heads turn to look at teenagers with tattoos and body piercing, people with hearing impairments signing, those using wheelchairs. It is a fact of life that looking different gets attention. Staring has power and meaning only to the degree to which we give it meaning and power over our lives.

I gradually found that most people stare because they are unfamiliar with burn injuries and feel compassion and concern. Others are simply curious. A few stare because they are overwhelmed by such a traumatic injury, and the fewest stare because they are rude.

What we see depends on what we are looking for

The way we choose to interpret and perceive stares will influence our ability to cope with them. If we focus our attention on staring and perceive stares as evil and threatening, then that will be our experience. If, however, we diminish the importance of staring and interpret stares as a mild inconvenience, that will be our experience. Our interpretations and perceptions either defeat or enhance our social success.

Faulty assumptions

In his book *The Body Image Workbook* Thomas Cash states that it is flawed thinking to assume that, simply because they notice you, people will dislike you: "friendliness, kindness, and conversational skills" are "more influential than whatever might be different about your looks." Instead, the truth is that "you are the one noticing what you don't like about your appearance." Other people usually do not care because they are thinking about other things.

In the first months after my burn injury, I wore clothing to hide my injuries and continually looked to see if people were "looking" at me. People staring and seeing my scars became the focus of my attention, and I felt uncomfortable in social settings. I spent much of my energy worrying what others thought. Many burn survivors have reported the same behaviour.

Cash also points out that "first impressions don't always last" and "our initial reactions to someone's appearance are not frozen forever in our minds." A person may focus on a burn survivor's appearance initially. I consider this pretty normal. When I meet another burn survivor for the first time, I often take a few minutes to "get used to" the new and unique skin patterns I am seeing. After we have established a relationship, however, the burns become less important, and personal traits such as intelligence, humour, integrity, and sensitivity are the most defining characteristics. Often I forget exactly where a person's burns are located—which side of the face, which hand, etc. By strengthening our social skills, we can overcome the challenge of looking "different."

So what do I do?

Barbara Quayle has developed some simple strategies to help those with physical differences respond in a positive way to questions and staring. By practising these strategies, many burn survivors have become more comfortable in social settings. These techniques are easily taught to patients before discharge from hospital, and they should be part of the care plan for all burn survivors.

"STEPS"

If you find yourself being stared at, Barbara suggests standing up straight, looking directly into the person's eyes, smiling, and, with a friendly tone of voice, saying "Hi, how are you doing?" or "Hi, how's it going?" or even "Hi, great day, isn't it?" Looking at

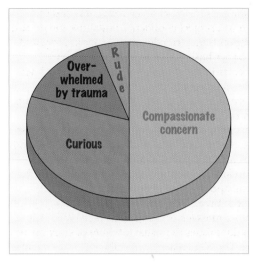

Reasons why people stare at burn survivors

"**You** are the one noticing what **you** don't like about your appearance."

"If you act like a victim, people will treat you like a victim."

B Quayle

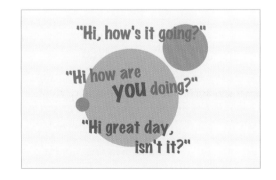

"Hi, how's it going?"

"Hi, how are **you** doing?"

"Hi, great day, isn't it?"

and speaking to the person shows social awareness and self confidence. When you project confidence and poise the person staring usually responds in a friendly manner, looks away, and goes on with his or her business. When a stare triggers a comfortable and confident response, the person is sometimes surprised and often a little embarrassed about staring. Remember, you are in control, not the person staring. Become conscious of your own behaviour.

If eye contact, smiling, and speaking seem like too much at first, simply "look 'em in the eye" and smile. Energy and warmth radiate from faces wearing smiles. People who smile at others have advantages in forming relationships because a smile often dispels the fear and apprehension of strangers. In new situations a smile can break barriers or end prejudicial judgments. It sends a message of being approachable and at ease. A smile also diminishes the visual intensity of scarring and skin discoloration. The STEPS acronym will help you remember to take control and not "act like a victim."

Another alternative is simply to ignore the person staring and go about your business. Sometimes this may be preferable if you are tired or not bothered by the stare. I never advocate reacting to staring with an angry response. Anger at others often hurts most the person who is angry. When you respond with anger it is usually out of fear and says more about you than the person staring. There will be times when you or a protective family member want to lash out verbally at someone staring, but being abusive does not reflect well on you or your family and may leave you feeling frustrated, resentful, and bitter.

"Rehearse your responses"

Another helpful technique that Barbara teaches is to be prepared for people's questions. Often burn survivors and their families feel awkward, uncomfortable, angry, or embarrassed when strangers ask questions about their burns. If survivors can develop a two or three sentence response to such questions and then practise this in privacy with family and healthcare professionals, they will have greater confidence in new social situations.

It first must be a conscious effort. Then, as you "rehearse your responses," you find it becomes second nature, and eventually you become proud of your positive attitude and how you handle social situations.

Healthcare professionals can help

It is the responsibility of healthcare professionals to discuss staring with burn survivors and their families before discharge. They need to know that some people will stare, ask questions; and helping them to practise specific strategies to use in public and in social situations can only assist them in making the successful transformation to a person who thrives after surviving a burn injury.

Competing interests: AA is executive director of the Phoenix Society for Burn Survivors.

The picture of a pressure garment is used with permission of Gottfried Medical.

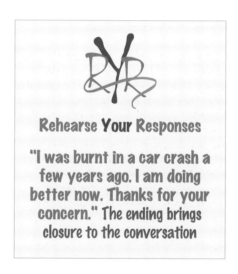

STEPS ©

BE SURE TO:

Use self talk (I can handle this confidently)

Speak in a friendly tone of voice

Look 'em in the eye

Posture - stand up straight

Wear a smile

Rehearse Your Responses

"I was burnt in a car crash a few years ago. I am doing better now. Thanks for your concern." The ending brings closure to the conversation

To learn more about support for burn survivors and to obtain articles by Barbara Kammerer Quayle and the Phoenix Society, visit the society's website at www.phoenix-society.org

Further reading
- Cash TF. *The body image workbook*. Oakland CA: New Harbinger Publications,1997
- Quayle BK. When people stare. *Burn Support News* 2001;2(summer).

Index

Notes: As burns are the subject of this book, all index entries refer to burns unless otherwise indicated. Page references in *italics* refer to figures, tables or boxed material.

acid burns 5
acrylic face mask, scar management 27, *27*
acute stage, psychological aspects 29–30, *30*
acute stress disorder, acute stage 29
airway
   control, inhalation injury 19
   management 10, *10*
   primary survey 10
   toilet, inhalation injury 20
airway burns 19–20, *20*
   see also inhalation injury
alcohol misuse 5
alkali burns 5
alloplastic materials, contraindications 25
Amnion, cost effectiveness *33*
analgesia
   first aid 7
   fixed dose schedule, effects *30*
   major burns 12
   rehabilitation 26
   see also pain control
antibiotics
   infection prevention 22
   inhalation injury 20
   minor burns 9, *9*
   topical, advantages/disadvantages 22
anxiety, prevalence 29
appearance, patient's attitudes 35–6
appearance of burn, depth *15*, 15
aseptic techniques, dressing changes 9
assessment of burn area, major burns 13
asthmatic patients, smoke inhalation 11

bacterial infection 21, *21*
   control 22
bitumen burns, facial injury *2*
blanching *see* capillary refill
blast lung 11
bleeding test, burn depth *15*, 15
blisters, management 8, *8*, 12
blood gas analysis 10, 11
blood tests, major burns 11
bone grafts, tissue deficiency 25
breathing
   mechanical restriction 11
   mechanics, inhalation injury 26, *26*
   primary survey 10–11
bronchoscopy *11*, 19
burn disasters 33–4
   characteristics *33*
   disaster plan *33*, 33–4, *34*
   first aid *34*
   management principles *33*
burning process, halting 7
Burnshield 7, *7*
burns unit referral
   healing failure 16
   major burns 12
butane gas, abuse *2*

calcium gluconate 6
Candida, infection 21
capillary refill
   burn depth test *15*, 15
   deep partial thickness burn 17
carbonaceous particles, facial burn *10*
carbon monoxide 19
carboxyhaemoglobin 11
carboxyhaemoglobinaemia 11, *11*
cardiac monitoring, electrical injury 5
cardiovascular changes 4
care/management
   aims 2
   cost effective *33*
   major burns 2
   minor burns 8, *8*
   strategies, developing world 32–3
cartilage grafts, tissue deficiency 25
Cash T, *The Body Image Workbook* 36
causes, of burns 1, *1*
   developing countries 32, *32*
cement, burns 5
cerebral failure, intensive care
     management 20
cerebral oedema, fluid resuscitation 20
cerium nitrate-silver sulfadiazine 22
cervical spine, control 10
'Changing Faces' 31
chemical injuries *5*, 5–6, *6*
   eyes 6
   management 6
chest burns, breathing problems 11
children
   burn risk 1
   maintenance fluid 14, *14*
   non-accidental injury 6, *6*
   scar contracture 24
   urinary output measurement 12
chromic acid burn, treatment 6
circulation, primary survey 11
circumferential burns 11
   surgery indication 14, *14*
cleaning, minor burns 8
cling film
   acute major burns 12
   first aid cover 7, *7*
clothing
   burning process 7
   burns risk 32, *32*
coagulation zone 4
Coban (compression glove) 27
codeine, contraindications 26
cognitive changes, intensive care unit 29
colloid infusion 13, 14
composite grafts 25
compression glove *27*
concomitant injuries
   major burns 11
   minor burns 8

Index

contact burns 5
  hot iron *5*
  non-accidental 6
  radiator *2*
contractures *see* scar contracture
cooking, developing world 32, *32*
cooling of burns 7
coping strategies 36
cost effectiveness, burn treatment 33
counselling
  peer 31
  psychological 30
critical stage, psychological aspects 29
crystalloid, maintenance 14
cultured epithelial autografts 18

death, inhalation injury 19
deep dermal burn 18, *18*
  definition 15
deep partial thickness burn 17
depression, prevalence 29
depth of burns
  assessment 14–15, *15*
    algorithm *18*
    estimation 15, *15*
  classification 15
  diagram *15*
  progression 27
  varying 16–18
developing countries, burns in 32–3
  admissions, reporting 33
  care strategies 32–3, *33*
  epidemiology 32
  management problems 32, *32*
  risk factors 32
  treatment 33, *33*
dichromate salts burn, treatment 6
disasters *see* burn disasters
disfigurement, concerns 9
domestic electricity, injuries 5
donor tissue, burns reconstruction 24
'doughnut sign', non-accidental injury 6, *6*
dressings 18
  burn disasters 34
  changing 8, *8*
  cost effectiveness 33
  first aid 7, *7*
  Hypafix *16*, 16
  major burns 12
  minor burns *8*, 8–9
  specialist 8–9
  strike through 8
  TransCyte *17*
Duoderm 9

ECG, post-electrocution *5*
education
  burn prevention 3
  scar management 28
elastomer moulds, scar management 28
elderly
  burn risk 2
  contact burn risk 5
  major burn *18*
electrical injuries 5
  first aid treatment 7
  history information 10
  investigations *12*
electrocardiogram, post-electrocution *5*
endogenous healing, environment 17
endotracheal intubation, inhalation injury 19
epidermal burns, treatment 16
epilepsy, contact burns 5

erythema, burn area calculations 13
escharotomies, major burns 14, *14*
excision
  deep partial thickness burn 17
  full thickness burns 17
  healthy tissue *17*
  major burns 18
  timing 17
exercise
  rehabilitation 26, *26, 28*
  see also physiotherapy
exposure of patient 11
extremity burns, circumferential 11
eye injuries, chemicals 6

facial burns
  carbonaceous particles *10*
  minor 9, *9*
family involvement, psychological recovery 29
Fire kills campaign *3*
  safety tips 3
fire safety 3
fireworks, burns risk 32, *32*
first aid 7
  burn disasters *34*
Flamazine 8, 9, *9*
  contraindications 12
flame injury 5
  burns various depths 16
flaps, burns reconstruction 24–5
flash burn 5
  vs high tension burn *5*
fluid resuscitation 12, 13–14
  aim 13
  airway burns 19
  cerebral oedema 20
  children 14, *14*
  colloid infusion 13, 14
  end point 14, *20*
  examples *14*
  fresh frozen plasma 14
  Hartman's solution 14
  high tension electrical injuries 14
  kidney failure 20
  maintenance crystalloid 14
  Parkland formula *see* Parkland
    formula
follow up
  minor burns 9
  outpatient, rehabilitation 28
fresh frozen plasma 14
full thickness burns 18
  black patient *15*
  definition 15
  treatment 17
fungal infection 21, *21*

Gamgee pads 34
Glasgow coma scale, major burns 11
grafting
  bacterial colonisation 21
  cultured epithelial autografts 18
  deep partial thickness burn 17
  full thickness burns 17
  major burns 18
  persistent mesh pattern *17*
  temporary coverings 17–18
  timing 17
  tissue deficiency 25
  types 17
Granuflex 9
grief 30
guilt, concerns 9

hand burns, first aid cover 7
Hartman's solution 14
healed burns, characteristics 9
healing failure, burns unit referral 16
healthcare professionals
    disaster plan *33*, 33–4
    non-accidental injury 6
    support 37
heart failure, intensive care management 20
herpes simplex infection 21
high tension electrical burns 5
    fluid resuscitation 14
    vs flash burn *5*
hospitals, disaster plan *33*, 33–4
hot gas inhalation 10
hydrocolloids, scar management *28*
hydrofluoric acid 5–6
Hypafix dressings *16*, 16
hyperaemia zone 4
hypermetabolic response 20, *20*
hypertrophic scarring 16, 27
    appearance *16, 27*
    therapy 9
hypoperfusion 13
hypovolaemia 11
hypoxia, fluid loss 13

illnesses, minor burns associated 8
immobilisation, rehabilitation 27, *27*
immunological changes, burn injuries 4
incidence, of burns 1, *1*, 32
India, burns incidence 32
infection 21–2
    causative agents *21*, 21–2
    common site 21
    contributory factors 21
    diagnosis 22
    pathogenesis 21
    prevention 22
    signs 21–2, *22*
    sites *21*
    treatment/control 22
inhalation injury
    airway control 19
    airway toilet 20
    breathing mechanics 26, *26*
    death 19
    diagnosis 19
    fluid resuscitation 19
    intensive care management 19–20
    investigations *12*
    key clinical points *20*
    lung insult mechanisms 19, *19*
    pathophysiology 19, *19*
    rehabilitation 26
    signs 10, *10*
    smoke 11
    treatment 19, 20, 26
    ventilatory strategies *20*
    warning signs 19, *19*
inotropic drug use 20
intensive care management *19*, 19–21
    airway burns *see* inhalation injury
    monitoring 20
    nutrition 20–1
    psychological aspects 29
intravenous access 11
intubation
    considerations 10
    inhalation injury 19
investigation, major burns 12
irons, contact burn *5*
itching 9, *9*

Jackson's burn zones 4, *4*
Jelonet *8*
    alternative 9
    minor burns 8, *8*
joints, scar contracture 24

keloid scarring 27
kerosene pressure stoves, burns risk 32, *32*
kidney failure, intensive care management 20

legislation, burn prevention 3
local response, burn injuries 4
lorazepam 30
Lund and Browder chart 13, *13*
lymphatic system, oedema reduction 26

mafenide 22
major burns 10–15
    aims of care *2*
    analgesia 12
    assessment of burn area 13
    assessment of burn depth *see* depth
        of burns
    blood tests 11
    care (steps) *2*
    concomitant injuries 11, 12
    definition 10
    dressings 12
    elderly patient *18*
    escharotomies 14, *14*
    fluid resuscitation *see* fluid resuscitation
    history, key points 10, *10*
    initial assessment 10, *10*
    investigation 12, *12*
    morphine 12
    neurological disability 11
    oxygen treatment 10
    primary survey 10–12, *11*
    prognosis 2–3
    referral to burns unit 12, *12*
    resuscitation 3, 13–15
    surgery 18
management of burns *see* care/
    management
massage, scar management *28*
Mepitel 9
meshed graft 17, *17*
metabolic changes, burn injuries 4
methicillin resistant *Staphylococcus aureus* 22
minor burns 8–9
    associated illness/injuries 8
    cleaning the wound 8
    dressings 8–9
    facial 9
    follow up 9
    outpatient treatment 8, *8*
mobility preservation, Hypafix dressings 16
moisturisers, scar management *28*
morphine, major burns 12
mortality 1, 21
    factors affecting 2–3, *3*
movement, rehabilitation 26, *26*, 28
MRSA 22
myoglobinuria *20*

narcotics, rehabilitation 26
National Burn Care Review, referral 12
neck contracture, release *24*
net dressing, minor burns 8, *8*
Netelast, minor burns 8, *8*
neurological disability, major burns 11
nightmares 30
non-accidental injury 6, *6*

Index

nutrition
  hypermetabolic response 20
  intensive care management 20–1
  tube feeding 21

occupational therapy, burns reconstruction 24
oedema
  cerebral, fluid resuscitation 20
  facial 9
  management, rehabilitation 26–7
opiates
  background pain 30
  first aid 7
  see also pain control
organ failure, oxygen treatment 19
oropharynx, inspection 10
outpatient follow up, rehabilitation 28
outpatient treatment, minor burns 8
oxygen treatment
  airway burns 19
  carboxyhaemoglobinaemia 11
  hyperbaric 11
  major burns 10

pain control
  background pain 30
  effects of fixed dose 30
  non-pharmacological 29, 30
  psychological aspects 30
  rehabilitation 26
  see also analgesia
palmar surface, burn area calculations 13
Parkland formula 13–14, 14
  cost effectiveness 33, 33
partial thickness burns, definition 15
pathophysiology of burn injuries 4–6
patient's perspective 35–7
  appearance, attitudes 35–6
  coping strategies 36
  facing the world 35
  staring see staring
  see also psychosocial aspects
patient support 9
patient-surgeon relationship 24
penetrating injuries, lungs 11
persistent mesh pattern 17
photographic workup 24
physical problems, rehabilitation 31
physiotherapy
  burns reconstruction 24
  exercise 26, 26, 28
  minor burns 9
pigmented skin, burn assessment 13
plasma, fresh frozen, fluid resuscitation 14
pneumonia, risk factors 21
polyvinyl chloride film see cling film
positive expiratory pressure device 26
post-traumatic stress disorder 29
premorbid psychopathology 30
pressure garments
  burns reconstruction 24
  scar management 27
prevention of burns 3
  developing countries 32–3
primary survey, major burns 10–12
  algorithm 11
prostheses, inflatable 25
pruritus 9, 9
pseudomonal colonisation, grafted burn 21
Pseudomonas infection, treatment 9
psychosocial aspects 29–31
  acute stage 29–30, 30
  pain control 30

prevalence of disorders 29
problems during rehabilitation 31, 31
rehabilitation see rehabilitation
resuscitative stage 29, 29
supportive treatments 29, 30, 31
see also patient's perspective
pulmonary infection 21
pulmonary insult, lower airway burns 19, 19
pulse oximetry 11
  carbon monoxide toxicity 19

Quayle BK 35

radiator, contact burn 2
reconstruction 23–5
  consultation/visit 24
  deficiency of tissue 25
  essentials 24
  flaps 24–5
  patient-surgeon relationship 24
  photographic workup 24
  release neck contracture 24
  scar contracture and release 23
  skin 27
  skin expansion 25
  surgical procedures 24–5
  techniques 23, 25
  timing 23, 23
  unstable burn scars 24
  Z-plasties 25, 25
referrals see burns unit referral
rehabilitation 26–8
  follow up 28
  immobilisation 27
  inhalation injury 26
  movement/exercise 26, 26, 28
  oedema management 26–7
  pain control 26
  physical problems 31
  psychosocial problems 31, 31
  scar management see scar(s), management
  see also reconstruction
respiratory changes, burn injuries 4
restraint marks, non-accidental injury 6
resuscitation
  fluid see fluid resuscitation
  major burns 3
  not resuscitating, decision 3
resuscitation effects, Jackson's burn zones 4
resuscitative stage, psychological aspects 29, 29
risk groups 1–2
  compromising factors 2
  contact burns 5
rule of nines, burn area calculations 13, 13

safety tips, Fire kills campaign 3
scalds 4–5
  appearance 1, 5
  deep dermal burn 18
  history information 10
  non-accidental 6, 6
  pathophysiology 4–5
  superficial 7, 8
scar(s) 27
  hypertrophic see hypertrophic scarring
  management 27–8
    garments 27, 27
    scar types 27
    team education 28
    techniques 28
  techniques to reduce reconstructive
    needs 23
  unstable, reconstruction 24

scar contracture *23*
    effect on joints 24
    reconstruction 24, *24*
    release *23*
self esteem 31
sensation, burn depth test *15*, 15
shaving, facial burns 9
silicon gel sheets, scar management *28*
silver nitrate 22
silver sulfadiazine 22
skin
    expansion method *25*
    grafts *see* grafting; *specific types*
    reconstruction 27
sleep disturbance 30
smoke inhalation 11
smoking, blood gas analysis 10
social services, non-accidental injury 6
split skin grafts 17, *17*
    donor sites 17
staphylococcal infections *21*
staring
    causes *36*
    coping strategies 36–7
    patient's perspective 36–7
    professional help 37
    situation control 36–7
stasis zone 4
STEPS, situation control 36–7
streptococcal cellulitis *21*
streptococcal infection 21
strike through, dressing 8
substance abuse
    butane gas *2*
    contact burns 5
sulphuric acid burn *5*
sunburn, treatment 9
sun protection, scar management 28
superficial burn, definition 15
superficial dermal burn 18
    definition 15
superficial partial thickness burns 16, 18

supportive treatments 29, 30, 31
surgery
    infection prevention 22
    timing 17–18
    see also grafting; reconstruction
systemic response, burn injuries 4, *4*

tar burns, first aid treatment 7
TENS, pain control 26
The Body Image Workbook 36
thermal injuries 4–5
topical creams, indications 8
transcutaneous electrical nerve stimulation 26
TransCyte 17
transportation, disaster plan 34
treatment *see* care/management
triage, burn disasters 34
tube feeding 21

ultrasound, scar management *28*
unmeshed graft, applications 17
urinary output measurement, major burns 12, 14
urine output, kidney failure 20

vasoconstriction 20
ventilation
    after inhalational injury 19, 26
    carboxyhaemoglobinaemia 11
    smoke inhalation 11
    strategies *20*
viral infection *21*, 21–2

Wallace rule of nines, burn area calculations 13, *13*
washing, Hypafix dressings 16
water, burn cooling 7
work, return to 31
wound
    biopsy 22
    infection signs 8

zones of burn 4, *4*
Z-plasties, burns reconstruction 25, *25*